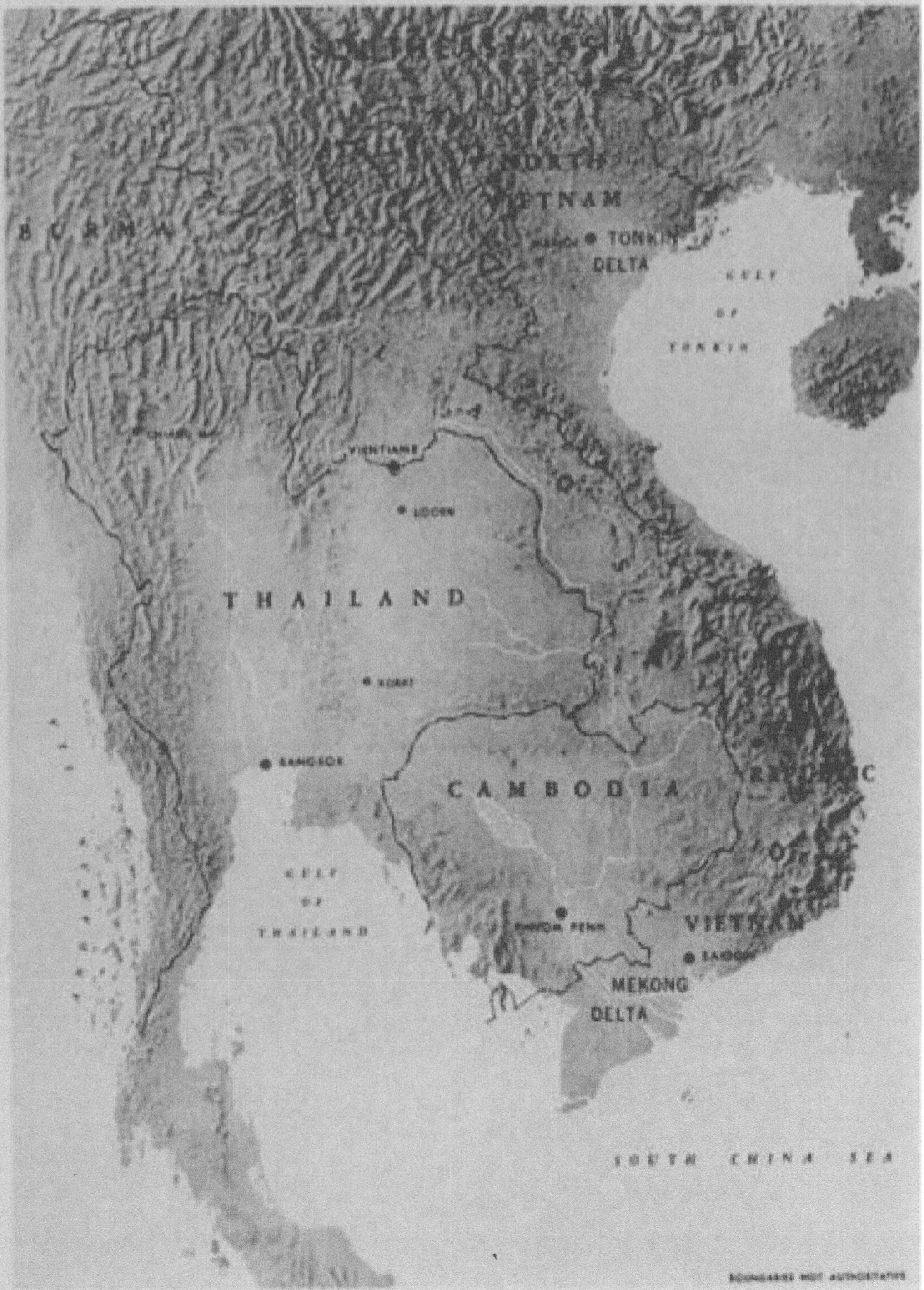
TONKIN
DELTA
GULF
OF
TONKIN
VIENTIANE
UDORN
THAILAND
KORAT
BANGKOK
CAMBODIA
GULF
OF
THAILAND
PHNOM PENH
SAIGON
MEKONG
DELTA
SOUTH CHINA SEA
BOUNDARIES NOT AUTHORITATIVE

VIETNAM STUDIES

MEDICAL SUPPORT OF THE U.S. ARMY IN VIETNAM 1965–1970

by

Major General Spurgeon Neel

DEPARTMENT OF THE ARMY

WASHINGTON, D.C., 1991

Library of Congress Catalog Card Number: 72-600264

First Printed 1973—CMH Pub 90-16

For sale by the Superintendent of Documents, U.S. Government Printing Office
Washington, D.C. 20402

Foreword

The United States Army has met an unusually complex challenge in Southeast Asia. In conjunction with the other services, the Army has fought in support of a national policy of assisting an emerging nation to develop governmental processes of its own choosing, free of outside coercion. In addition to the usual problems of waging armed conflict, the assignment in Southeast Asia has required superimposing the immensely sophisticated tasks of a modern army upon an underdeveloped environment and adapting them to demands covering a wide spectrum. These involved helping to fulfill the basic needs of an agrarian population, dealing with the frustrations of antiguerrilla operations, and conducting conventional campaigns against well-trained and determined regular units.

As this assignment nears an end, the U.S. Army must prepare for other challenges that may lie ahead. While cognizant that history never repeats itself exactly and that no army ever profited from trying to meet a new challenge in terms of the old one, the Army nevertheless stands to benefit immensely from a study of its experience, its shortcomings no less than its achievements.

Aware that some years must elapse before the official histories will provide a detailed and objective analysis of the experience in Southeast Asia, we have sought a forum whereby some of the more salient aspects of that experience can be made available now. At the request of the Chief of Staff, a representative group of senior officers who served in important posts in Vietnam and who still carry a heavy burden of day-to-day responsibilities has prepared a series of monographs. These studies should be of great value in helping the Army develop future operational concepts while at the same time contributing to the historical record and providing the American public with an interim report on the performance of men and officers who have responded, as others have through our history, to exacting and trying demands.

All monographs in the series are based primarily on official records, with additional material from published and unpublished secondary works, from debriefing reports and interviews with key participants, and from the personal experience of the author. To facilitate security clearance, annotation and detailed bibliography have been omitted from the published version: a fully documented account with bibliography is filed with the Office of the Chief of Military History.

Major General Spurgeon Neel is especially qualified to write a study of the Medical Department support of the U.S. Army in Vietnam. Not only is General Neel one of the most decorated Medical Corps officers presently on active duty, but he is also a specialist in a variety of military-medical disciplines. A Senior Flight Surgeon, Senior Parachutist, and Senior Gliderist, he is the Army's leading authority on Aviation Medicine. This, coupled with his clinical expertise in the specialty of Preventive Medicine, and his broad and varied command and staff experience, place him in the forefront of those who can write authoritatively of the Medical Department's role in Vietnam.

General Neel has served two tours of duty in Vietnam, in positions of extreme responsibility, which enabled him to participate in the major decisions regarding medical support of the Allied Forces. From 1966 to 1967, he was the USMACV Surgeon and Senior Adviser to General Westmoreland. Later, 1968 to 1969, he returned to Vietnam and served initially as CG, 44th Medical Brigade, and Surgeon, USARV, and subsequently, as Surgeon, USMACV, and principal medical adviser to General Abrams. Upon his return to CONUS, General Neel was nominated Deputy Surgeon General, Department of the Army, the position in which he has served since 1 October 1969.

In addition to this study, General Neel is the author of some 33 articles which have been published in leading professional journals in this country and abroad. His present work constitutes a candidly expressed authentic overview of the Medical Department's experiences in Vietnam which should be of considerable interest and benefit to all students of this period in our history.

VERNE L. BOWERS
Major General, USA
The Adjutant General

Washington, D.C.
15 August 1972

Preface

General Westmoreland's request that I prepare a monograph setting forth activities of the Medical Department in support of the U.S. Army in Vietnam, for the years 1965–1970, was most welcome since I had but recently returned from a second tour in Vietnam during which time I had held the positions of Surgeon, U.S. Army, Vietnam (USARV) and Surgeon, U.S. Military Assistance Command, Vietnam (USMACV).

The purpose of this monograph is to provide a meaningful overview of significant medical problems encountered and decisions made, of achievements and mistakes, and of lessons learned in Vietnam. The hope is that this study will provide a source of information for future planning, pending the writing of the definitive history of the Army Medical Department in Vietnam.

Emphasis is placed on perspective rather than detail. In addition to describing the events that occurred, I have sought to explain why decisions were made and specific actions taken. Purely technical medical considerations are not within the scope of this monograph. An evaluation of the health of the command and the care provided to battle casualties is made within an operational context. The absence of more detail on the magnificent support provided by medical elements of the U.S. Air Force and U.S. Navy to U.S. Army medical operations is the result of the need for brevity rather than lack of appreciation.

In planning the outline of this monograph, I gave consideration to the duties, experiences, and actions which make up the total of Medical Department support of the Army. I decided to concentrate on the major subdivisions of the medical service rather than deal with all aspects superficially.

This study tells the story of the Army Medical Department in Vietnam. Hopefully, this experience will provide a basis for those who must evaluate our current doctrine and organization and for those who will be responsible for planning the medical support of future operations.

It is with no little pride that one can say that the facts give concrete evidence of the magnificent job done by the men and women who comprise the Army Medical Department in Vietnam.

In conclusion, I wish to acknowledge the efforts of the many contributors who made this monograph possible. This study was, as can well be imagined, no one-man job. I am grateful to the members of the various directorates and offices of the Office of The Surgeon General who provided me with material, and especially appreciative of the efforts of the members of The Historical Unit, U.S. Army Medical Department, for their technical assistance in the preparation and editing of the manuscript.

SPURGEON NEEL, M.D.
Major General, U.S. Army
Deputy Surgeon General

Washington, D.C.
15 August 1972

Contents

Tables

Charts

Maps

Illustrations

Illustrations are from Department of Defense files.

Introduction

Full understanding of medical operations in Vietnam requires some appreciation of the nature of the country and of the war that has been waged there.

The Republic of Vietnam lies entirely within the Tropics. Saigon is halfway around the world from Washington, D.C. There is a 12-hour difference in time between the two cities. The nearest off-shore U.S. hospital is almost 1,000 miles away at Clark Air Force Base in the Philippines. The nearest logistical support base is about 1,800 miles away in Okinawa. The nearest complete hospital center is in Japan, some 2,700 miles distant. Patients being evacuated to the United States must travel some 7,800 miles to reach Travis Air Force Base in California, or almost 9,000 miles to reach Andrews Air Force Base, near Washington, D.C.

Because of these distances, even with modern air transport, the need for self-sufficiency in the zone of operations is greater than that normally required within a combat zone. This fact is reflected by a higher ratio of combat service support troops (including medical) to combat troops than is normally provided in more conventional situations. Vietnam is actually a combat zone combined with the advanced section of a communications zone. The distance of Vietnam from the logistical support base also has an adverse effect on the efficiency and morale of troops newly arrived in-country.

Since 1954 Vietnam has been divided like Korea. North of the 17th parallel and Ben Hai River lies Communist North Vietnam and south is the free Republic of Vietnam. South Vietnam has a typically tropical climate of two seasons: hot and dry and hot and rainy. South Vietnam's continuously high temperature and humidity, its monsoon climate, and perennial dust-rain cycle have an obvious impact upon the types of diseases to be expected and upon the provision of medical care.

The majority of tropical diseases are both endemic and epidemic in South Vietnam. The high ambient temperature and humidity adversely affect the efficiency and health of U.S. troops fighting in this area, and the medical personnel supporting them. These also make it difficult to preserve and maintain medical supplies and sophisticated medical equipment. South Vietnam's terrain, with its waterways and jungles, impedes patient evacuation and supply distribution, even without the interference of combat operations.

The Republic of Vietnam is less than half the size of California and long and narrow like that state. It stretches some 700 miles from north to south, and is only 125 miles at its widest. It occupies the eastern and southern part of the Indochinese Peninsula in Southeast Asia, and borders the South China Sea and the Gulf of Siam. Near neighbors to the west are Laos, Cambodia, and Thailand. Several good ports along the eastern shore form the bases for logistical support of combat forces deployed inland and, in turn, affect the disposition of medical installations. The peninsular nature of Vietnam facilitates the employment of U.S. Navy hospital ships offshore in the South China Sea.

The conflict in Vietnam is a limited war as well as a counterinsurgency operation with the essential characteristics of both. There has been no ground or air confrontation between major powers. There has been no enemy aerial bombing of friendly troops, and artillery and rocket bombardment has been sporadic. The tour of duty in Vietnam is limited to 12 months, and forces in Vietnam enjoy a relatively high priority for all U.S. military resources.

The Republic of Vietnam is a sovereign nation. U.S. forces are there at the invitation of the host government to help maintain this sovereignty. Economic, political, and sociological factors affect the conduct of military operations. Vietnam, like most developing nations, suffers a paucity of medical resources. Through various medical civil assistance programs, the Army Medical Department has helped achieve national objectives in all facets of stability operations. Similarly, medical advice provided to the medical department of the Republic of Vietnam Armed Forces, has played a vital role in increasing the department's competence, capability, and self-reliance.

Guerrilla and terrorist operations throughout the country, interspersed with sporadic organized unit assaults against cities and military bases, characterize enemy tactics. There is no defined main line of resistance. The battle has been for popular support and stability, rather than for terrain, per se. Casualties occur anywhere at any time. There are no secure ground lines of communications outside of base areas.

The conflict has involved highly mobile, small tactical units, and has not been a war of mass movement of major military formations. Search and destroy operations by small units from relatively secure base areas and for relatively short periods of time have been characteristic. There has been a high reliance on organic Army air mobility for the conduct and support of these operations.

The Army Medical Department's deployments and procedures have reflected these tactical realities. Treatment facilities located in base areas receive casualties by air from operating combat elements. Because there was no need to move frequently, it was practicable to construct semipermanent medical facilities, thereby allowing the utilization of more sophisticated equipment and providing a general upgrading of the level of medical care.

At the beginning of 1965, the USMACV advisory effort was predominant, almost to the exclusion of all other U.S. Army medical support functions in Vietnam. There were some 20,000 U.S. troops in-country receiving medical support from two 100-bed hospitals (the U.S. Navy Hospital in Saigon and the U.S. Army's 8th Field Hospital in Nha Trang), plus some miscellaneous small medical detachments providing air evacuation and dispensary, laboratory, dental, and veterinary services.

The planning and implementing of medical support for the tactical and logistical buildup of Army forces in Vietnam have been challenging tasks. Many imponderables existed, mostly related to the nature of the country, the nature of the conflict, and the nature of the medical problems to be met. Estimates and plans based upon previous experience had to be modified to fit the unique situations in Vietnam as valid information was developed and a highly effective medical service created.

MEDICAL SUPPORT OF THE U.S. ARMY
IN VIETNAM, 1965–1970

CHAPTER I

The Medical Command Structure

Formal U.S. military assistance to the Republic of Vietnam may be traced to the signing of the Pentalateral Agreement in 1950, a multinational Mutual Defense Assistance Treaty for Indochina. The American contribution to the defense of the Southeast Asian sovereignties was nominal for several years thereafter, as reflected by the fact that at no time during the next decade did U.S. military personnel in Vietnam number more than 1,000. Most of the U.S. support effort took the form of materiel and supplies, distributed to the South Vietnamese government through MAAGV (Military Assistance Advisory Group, Vietnam), a small logistics and training organization. However, in November 1961, mounting support by North Vietnam of guerrilla activities in the South led President John F. Kennedy to conclude that, if the South Vietnamese democracy were to be preserved, a much larger commitment of U.S. military personnel in support of the RVNAF (Republic of Vietnam Armed Forces) would be required.

The consequences of the President's decision were immediately manifest. By the end of 1961, the number of U.S. military personnel in Vietnam had quadrupled. Slightly more than 4,000 men were assigned as military advisers to the RVNAF, to staff officers at MAAGV headquarters, or to a rapidly increasing number of support units. With the arrival of additional Special Forces and logistical detachments in the first 2 months of 1962, the magnitude of the U.S. military role in Vietnam became clear. To provide centralized command and control for these growing combat advisory and support forces, USMACV (U.S. Military Assistance Command, Vietnam), a joint command under CINCPAC (Commander in Chief, Pacific), was officially established on 8 February 1962. Named as the first COMUSMACV (Commander, U.S. Military Assistance Command, Vietnam) was Lieutenant General Paul D. Harkins, whose grade was indicative of the strength of the expanding American commitment.

Closely related to the buildup of American combat, combat advisory, and support forces was the development of the U.S. medical service structure in Vietnam. Based on anticipated troop lists, initial medical support requirements were set in December 1961, shortly after President Kennedy's decision to increase the level of American support to the RVNAF. These requirements included one field hospital of 100-bed capacity, with four attached medical detachments to provide specialty care but to be totally dependent on the hospital for administration and logistics, and one helicopter ambulance detachment to provide evacuation capability to the treatment facility.

Over-all planning and guidance for the deployment of all incoming units became the responsibility of CINCPAC under the direction of the Joint Chiefs of Staff and the Department of Defense. Logistical support responsibility was subsequently isolated and delegated to USARYIS (U.S. Army, Ryukyu Islands), a subordinate command of USARPAC (U.S. Army, Pacific). Logistical support of the medical units committed to Vietnam would become a major responsibility of the USARYIS surgeon's headquarters.

Medical Service During the Advisory Years

The field hospital recommended for deployment in December 1961 was to become operational in April of the following year. In the interim, however, arriving Army units, primarily transportation companies, could not be left without any form of medical service. During January and February 1962, three small medical detachments, each attached to a transportation company, disembarked in South Vietnam. Each provided, on an area basis, limited dispensary and general medical care for the units to which they were attached, as well as for all other U.S. personnel in their area.

To co-ordinate logistical and administrative support for the increasing number of U.S. Army personnel and units, USARYIS Support Group (Provisional) was established. On 24 February 1962, its medical section, comprised of one plans and operations officer and a chief clerk, both temporarily reassigned from the medical section of the 9th Logistical Command in Thailand, initiated medical activities in Vietnam. Through March, the medical section concentrated on assessing the capabilities of Army medical units in Vietnam, recommending to USARPAC through USARYIS headquarters that preventive medicine and veterinary food inspection detachments be sent from the United States to the theater of operations. Those requirements were subsequently corroborated by Major General Achilles L. Tynes, MC, USARPAC chief surgeon, and Colonel Thomas P. Caito, MSC, chief of his plans and operations division during a prolonged visit both made to Southeast Asia between 30 March and 1 May 1962.

However, the medical section would not see the fruition of its efforts as a staff office of the USARYIS Support Group (Provisional) headquarters. On 1 April 1962, the temporary USARYIS Support Group was redesignated USASGV (U.S. Army Support Group, Vietnam), and placed under the command and control of General Harkins as

COMUSMACV. The mission of the USASGV medical section was now clarified: to advise the USASGV commander and his staff on matters pertaining to the medical, dental, and veterinary services of the command, and to supervise all technical aspects of those services.

Less than 3 weeks later, on 18 April 1962, the 8th Field Hospital became operational at Nha Trang, assuming responsibility for the hospitalization of all authorized U.S. military personnel, dependents, and civilians living or stationed in Vietnam. A second responsibility allotted the 8th Field Hospital was that it act as a central medical supply point for all Army medical units in Vietnam, a duty for which the facility was ill-prepared and grossly understaffed.

Concurrently, the hospital commander, Lieutenant Colonel Carl A. Fischer, MC, became also the USASGV surgeon, staff adviser to the Commanding Officer, USASGV, on all Army medical activities in Vietnam. (*Chart 1*) As surgeon, Colonel Fischer also headed the USASGV medical section, now expanded to include one Medical Service Corps officer acting as chief of section and two enlisted men. Physically separated by some 200 miles from USASGV headquarters, Colonel Fischer made frequent trips from Nha Trang to Saigon to insure that all necessary action required of his medical section was accomplished. In addition, he had to utilize clerical personnel assigned to the 8th Field Hospital in performing those duties required of him as USASGV surgeon. Both arrangements proved unsatisfactory, prompting Colonel Fischer to request a change in the table of distribution based on AR 40–1; a change which, if approved, would have placed a full-time surgeon in USASGV headquarters. He further reported that, as of 31 December 1962, one of the major problems he faced as hospital commander was that of insufficient personnel in his headquarters section, leading to the absence of a "cohesive, balanced organization to accomplish the administrative and logistics burdens of attached units."

By the end of December, the number of detachments offering area medical coverage for U.S. forces, all obtaining their medical supplies through the 8th Field Hospital, had doubled. (*Map 1*) An even greater strain on the resources of that facility was created by attached units: two medical laboratories, three specialized surgical detachments, one segmented helicopter ambulance detachment, one dental detachment, one veterinary detachment, and one engineer detachment. While the veterinary detachment was headquartered in Saigon, all other units were totally dependent on the 8th Field Hospital for administration and logistics. The dual problems thus engendered—medical staffs too small to handle the administrative tasks demanded of them, and the physical separation of the USASGV surgeon from his medical section—would continue to plague the commanding officer of the 8th Field Hospital and his successors during the next 3 years.

Chart 1—Medical Command and Staff Structure, U.S. Army, Vietnam, 24 February 1962–1 April 1965

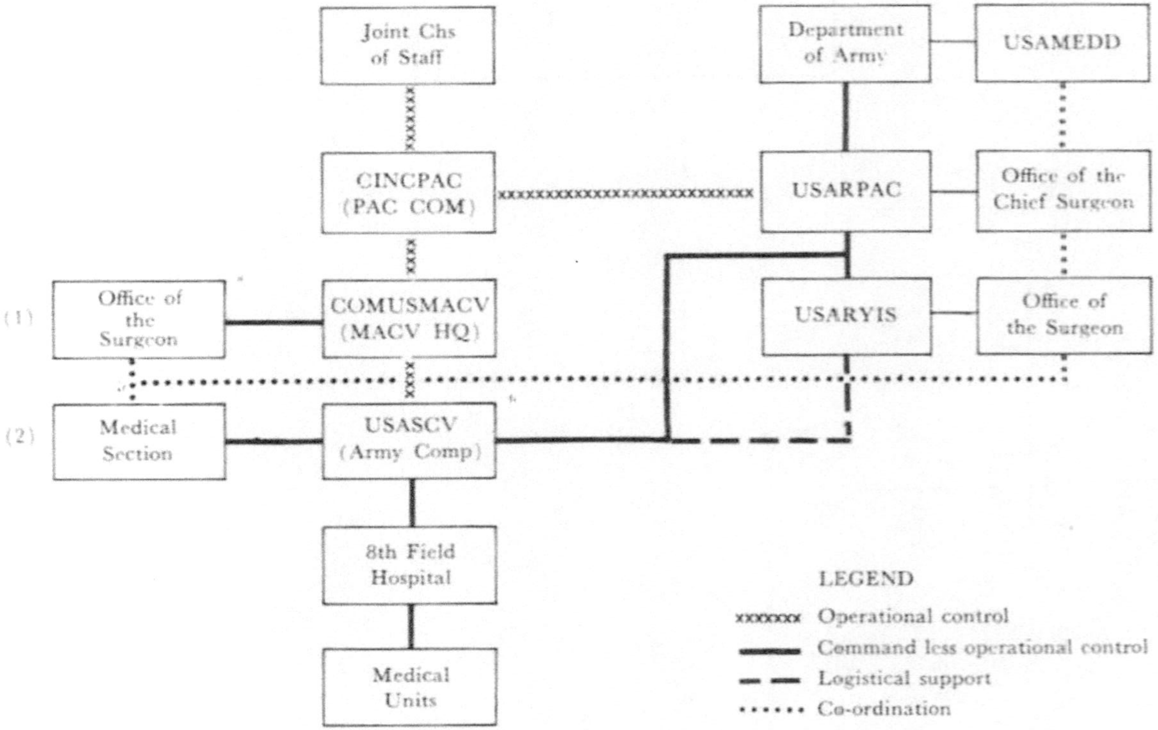

(1) Office of the Surgeon: MACV

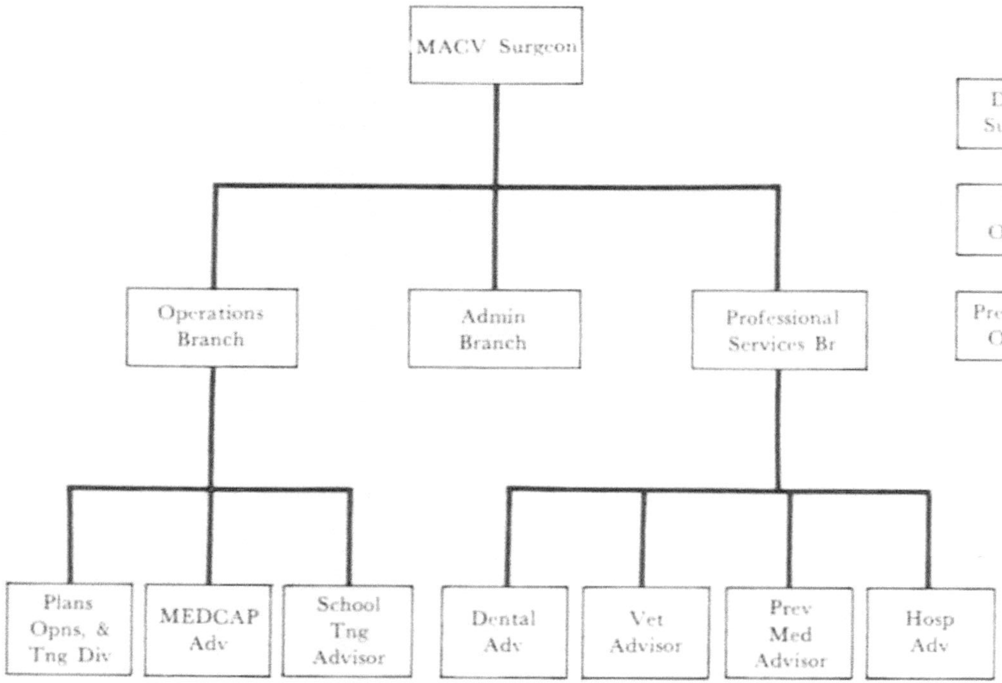

(2) Medical Section: USASCV

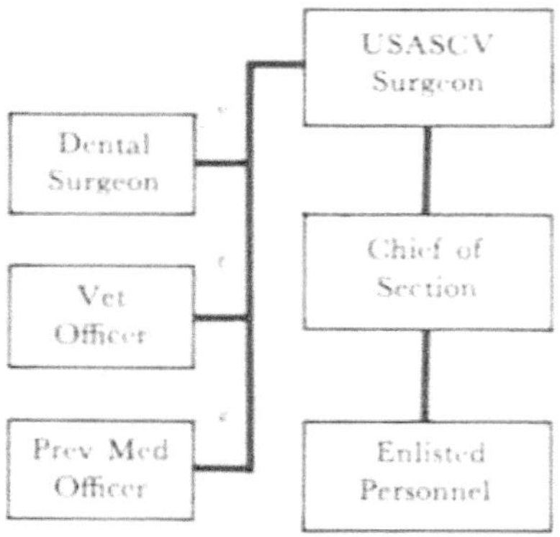

Although the opening of a Navy dispensary in Saigon in 1963 removed that city, as well as III and IV CTZ's (corps tactical zones) to the south, from the hospitalization responsibilities of the 8th Field Hospital, increasing numbers of casualties more than offset that relief. In the same year, USASGV was again redesignated, becoming USASCV (U.S. Army Support Command, Vietnam). Now removed from his direct command, General Harkins as COMUSMACV retained operational control over the lower headquarters. As the senior Army officer in Vietnam, however, he remained the Army component commander, while the Commanding General, USASCV, became deputy Army component commander. No benefits accrued to the USASCV medical section, however, and it remained understaffed and physically separated from the commanding officer of the 8th Field Hospital.

The Army medical structure in Vietnam remained essentially unchanged in 1964. The USASCV surgeon's medical section increased by one enlisted man; and while a dental surgeon, preventive medicine officer, and veterinarian were added to his staff, they too served in dual capacities and could contribute little to a reduction in the medical section's workload.

NOTES TO CHART 1

[a] Before the arrival of the 8th Field Hospital, administrative and logistical support for all Army medical units in Vietnam had been co-ordinated through the Office of the Surgeon, Headquarters, United States Military Assistance Command, Vietnam.

[b] USASCV was the acronym for the Army component headquarters in Vietnam from March 1963 through June 1965. Before 1963, that headquarters had been known as the USARYIS Support Group (Provisional) and, after 1 April 1962, as USASGV (United States Army Support Group, Vietnam).

[c] The staff structure of the Office of the Surgeon, Headquarters, MACV, as of 31 December 1964.

[d] The staff structure of the USASCV Medical Section as of 31 December 1964.

[e] The principal duty of the USASCV Dental Surgeon was Commanding Officer, 36th Medical Detachment (Dental Service), the command and control element for dental units.

[f] The principal duty of the USASCV Veterinary Officer was Commanding Officer, 4th Medical Detachment (Veterinary Food Inspection), the command and control element for veterinary units.

[g] The principal duty of the USASCV Preventive Medicine Officer was Commanding Officer, 20th Preventive Medicine Unit, the command and control element for preventive medicine units.

[h] The principal duty of the USASCV Surgeon was Commanding Officer, 8th Field Hospital, the senior medical organization and highest level headquarters for all nondivisional medical units in Vietnam.

[i] The plans and operations officer acting as chief of section, as well as the enlisted personnel under him, had originally constituted the Medical Section of the 9th Logistical Command, Thailand, whence they had been reassigned for temporary duty to South Vietnam.

Sources: (1) Medical Activities Report, Office of the Surgeon, Headquarters, Military Assistance Command, Vietnam, 1964. (2) Army Medical Service Activities Report, Medical Section, United States Army Support Command, Vietnam, 1964. (3) Army Medical Service Activities Report, Office of the Surgeon, Headquarters, United States Army, Vietnam, 1965.

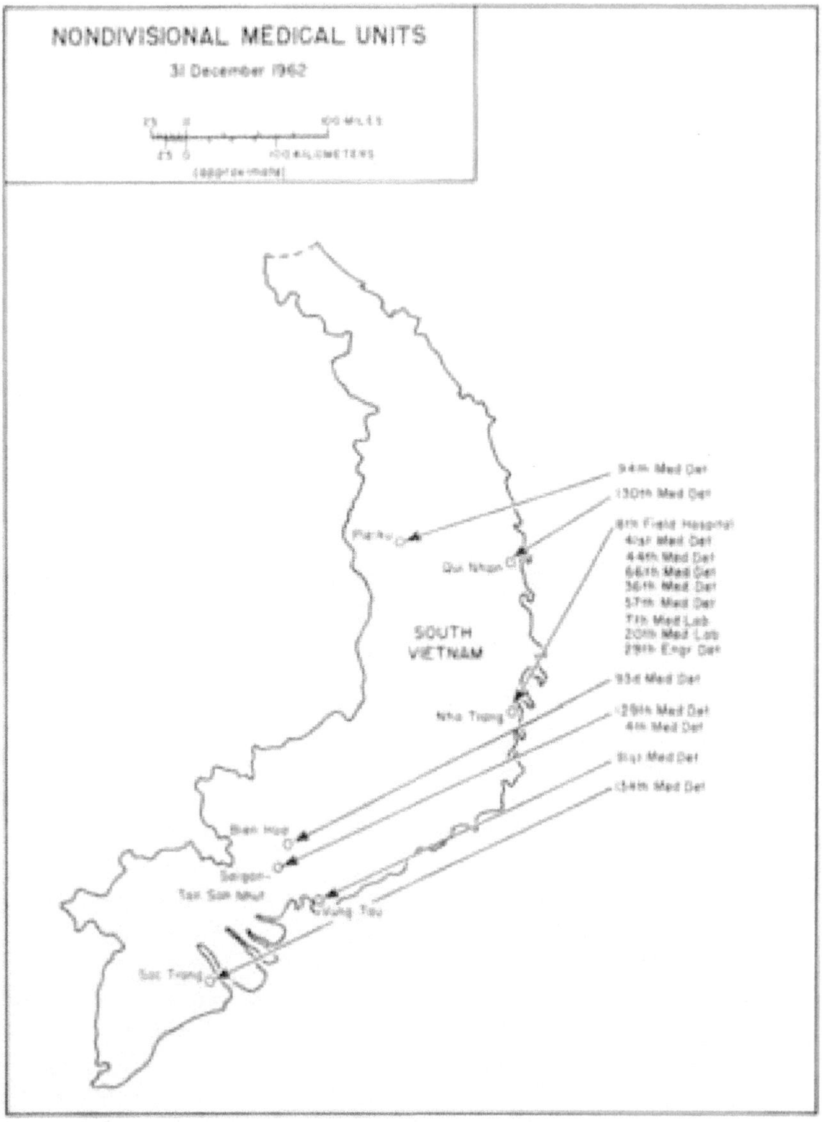

Map 1

Command and Staff Relationships During the Years of Military Commitment: 1965–67

Two American destroyers were attacked by North Vietnamese PT-boats on 2 and 4 August 1964, prompting the Gulf of Tonkin resolution. That action taken by Congress would lead to the direct commitment of the first major U.S. combat units in Vietnam. It would thrust General William C. Westmoreland, who had replaced General Harkins as

COMUSMACV shortly after the consolidation of MAAGV and USMACV headquarters in June 1964, into a position of international prominence; and it would be he who would supervise the massive buildup of U.S. forces in Vietnam over the next 4 years.

Medical Command Versus Logistical Command

As early as 1962, General Harkins had recognized the need for a centralized logistics organization in support of U.S. forces in South Vietnam. Again in 1964, COMUSMACV had recommended that a logistical command be promptly introduced in-country. Later in the year, the organization of that command was authorized, with responsibility for over-all joint logistical planning to reside in USMACV headquarters. The decision stipulated that support should be conducted on an area basis for all common supply and service activities, which in practice meant that the Army was to provide common-item support within II, III, and IV CTZ, plus any portion of I Corps in which major Army forces were deployed.

The doctrinal framework which justified the creation of a logistical command in Vietnam was COSTAR II, the second of two studies on combat service support of the Army. One of the outgrowths of the study was the directive that, when a field army was constituted, all logistical support was to be provided by FASCOM, a field army support command. Nondivisional medical service was placed under the Army support command.

The juxtaposition of two events (the decision of the Joint Chiefs of Staff to establish a centralized logistical command in Vietnam and the Gulf of Tonkin aftermath) made it only a matter of time before the U.S. Army would assume responsibility in South Vietnam for the distribution of supply items common to all military services, as well as for those used only by the Army.

On 1 April 1965, Headquarters, 1st Logistical Command, a field army support command and control element, was activated. In accordance with the policy of centralized logistical direction, four geographic support areas (roughly corresponding to CTZ's) were directly subordinated to that command. The 8th Field Hospital was removed from the direct command of USASCV headquarters and subordinated to the 1st Logistical Command. As senior medical officer in Vietnam, the hospital commander, Lieutenant Colonel (later Colonel) James W. Blunt, MC, now assumed a third hat: 1st Logistical Command surgeon and director of the command's medical section.

When Colonel Blunt activated the 1st Logistical Command medical section on 1 April, he was made responsible for providing the commander and his staff with necessary assistance and advice on all aspects of nondivisional medical support, to include veterinary and dental service, and medical supply. That proved an impossible task, since he remained both USASCV surgeon and commanding officer of the 8th Field Hospital. Colonel Blunt's dilemma was partially resolved with the interim appointment of a more junior Medical Corps officer, Major (later Lieutenant Colonel) Stuart A. Chamblin, Jr., as the 1st Logistical Command surgeon on 12 May. However, far more important changes in the structure of the Army medical service in Vietnam were imminent and would, for a time, reduce if not eliminate the problems faced by preceding commanding officers of the field hospital.

Consistent with current concepts, the USARPAC chief surgeon noted in his 1965 Annual Medical Activities Report: "Medical Service is an Army or area wide service and, as such, all medical support capability should be consolidated under one Medical Command." Prompting that statement were the recognized criticality of professional medical personnel, the unique characteristics of medical supply and maintenance, the constant demand for strong and effective preventive medicine and veterinary food inspection programs, and the requirement for medical support to be immediately responsive to the needs of the commander. A field hospital was completely unsuitable as a control element for a medical command encompassing units scattered through three CTZ's. Consequently, the 58th Medical Battalion was assigned to the 1st Logistical Command on 29 May, assuming command and control over nondivisional Army medical units in Vietnam. The battalion's commanding officer, Lieutenant Colonel (later Colonel) Edward S. Bres, Jr., MC, was simultaneously appointed 1st Logistical Command surgeon and director of its small organic medical planning staff.

With the appointment of Colonel Bres as 1st Logistical Command surgeon, the commanding officer of the 8th Field Hospital once again wore only two hats. However, the need for a full-time surgeon in the Army component headquarters had not diminished, but rather had become more pressing. The Department of the Army finally concurred in the oft-repeated demands of earlier USASCV surgeons, and on 29 June, authorized a table of distribution change adding a full-time surgeon, an administrative officer, and an additional enlisted man to the USASCV medical section. Ten days later, Lieutenant Colonel (later Colonel) Ralph E. Conant, MC, became the USASCV surgeon. Assigned no duties other than surgeon, he retained that post when USASCV was redesignated USARV (U.S. Army, Vietnam), on 20 July 1965.

The scope of the medical advisory effort at the field army level increased with the establishment of USARV as the highest command and control headquarters for all U.S. Army units in Vietnam. Reorganized in structure and expanded in size, the USASCV medical section was renamed the Office of the Surgeon, Headquarters, USARV. Staff supervision of a medical service supporting Army logistical operations had ceased to be a responsibility of the medical section when the 1st Logistical Command's medical section was activated. But on 20 July, that loss was more than offset with the assumption of staff responsibility for the health services of the entire Army medical structure in Vietnam, including unit, division, and army level medical service. Specifically, the USARV surgeon was given the mission of planning all USARV medical service, to be correlated at USARV headquarters with troop concentrations, logistical support areas, and the concept of tactical operations. Additional duties included preparing and co-ordinating broad medical policies, recommending assignments for medical personnel within USARV, maintaining medical records and statistics, and furnishing professional consultants to the command.

In the meantime, the 1st Logistical Command surgeon was coordinating the deployment and day-to-day operations of nondivisional medical units in Vietnam, units increasing in numbers from 11 in April to 60 by early fall. Just as the 8th Field Hospital had earlier proved inadequate as a command and control element, so now was Headquarters, 58th Medical Battalion, too small to handle the increasing volume of logistical, administrative, and support functions demanded by subordinate headquarters. On 18 August, Lieutenant Colonel Conant was replaced as USARV surgeon by Colonel Samuel C. Gallup, MC. On 25 October, the recently promoted Colonel Conant in turn replaced Colonel Bres as 1st Logistical Command surgeon. The reason for the replacement of Colonel Bres was soon apparent, for with the activation of the 43d Medical Group on 1 November, the 58th Medical Battalion ceased to be the senior army level medical unit in Vietnam. (*Chart 2*) Colonel Conant was the commanding officer of that medical group.

Although a subordinate medical headquarters, the 58th Medical Battalion continued to exercise major command and control responsibilities through 17 March 1966. The 43d Medical Group assumed the nondivisional medical service mission in II CTZ, and also exercised command and operational control over all nondivisional medical maintenance, laboratory, and helicopter units in Vietnam. The 58th Medical Battalion remained the command and control element for nondivisional units in III and IV CTZ's, and for all preventive medicine, dental, and veterinary units, until the 68th Medical Group became operational on 18 March 1966.

Command by the Medical Brigade

In December 1965, Lieutenant General Leonard D. Heaton, The Surgeon General, and General Westmoreland decided to send a medical brigade to Vietnam. Agreement had not been reached, however, on the level at which the brigade should be assigned. A month earlier, The Surgeon General visited Southeast Asia and, at that time, had concluded that the medical brigade should be made a major subordinate command of USARV headquarters, just as were the aviation and military police brigades and the engineer command. Shortly thereafter, Colonel (later Major General) Spurgeon Neel, MC, USMACV surgeon, had prepared a memorandum for General Westmoreland recommending that the medical brigade could most effectively support Army personnel in Vietnam if placed under the direct supervision of the USARV surgeon. Pointing out that medical service is an integrated function consisting of treatment, evacuation, and supply, Colonel Neel maintained that optimal medical service could only be achieved if directed solely by professional medical personnel. The interposition of an intermediate, nonmedical headquarters between responsible commanders and their medical resources could only reduce the quality of medical care available to troops. During the same interval, the USARPAC chief surgeon, Brigadier General (later Major General) Byron L. Steger, MC, had visited Vietnam and strongly recommended the release of medical service from logistical command and control.

The designated commanding officer of the medical brigade, Colonel (later Major General) James A. Wier, MC, nonetheless found that, upon his arrival in January, no decision as to the placement of his command had been made. Under the COSTAR II concept, medical service was visualized as a logistical service and, as such, belonged under FASCOM, the 1st Logistical Command. The FASCOM commanding general, Major General Charles W. Eifler, was unconvinced of the need for a medical brigade, preferring instead that medical groups be placed under the operational control of the commanding officers of each of his three area support commands. In that manner, General Eifler believed, all logistical support would be more responsive to the needs of the commanders of the two Field Force headquarters, and the mission of FASCOM best accomplished.

Since existing doctrine lent support to the position of General Eifler, Colonel Wier was made director of Medical Service and Supply on the General Staff of the FASCOM commanding general on 26 January 1966. Colonel Conant, who had previously occupied that position, was to remain 1st Logistical Command surgeon until the arrival of the medical brigade. In a March briefing attended by Major General (later Lieutenant General) John Norton, Deputy Commanding General, USARV, and General Eifler, Colonel Wier made a final attempt to have the medical brigade assigned directly to USARV headquarters, but to no avail. He succeeded only in persuading all concerned that the senior medical officer in Vietnam should be the USARV surgeon at the Army com-

Chart 2—Medical Command and Staff Structure, U.S. Army, Vietnam, 1 November 1965–17 February 1966

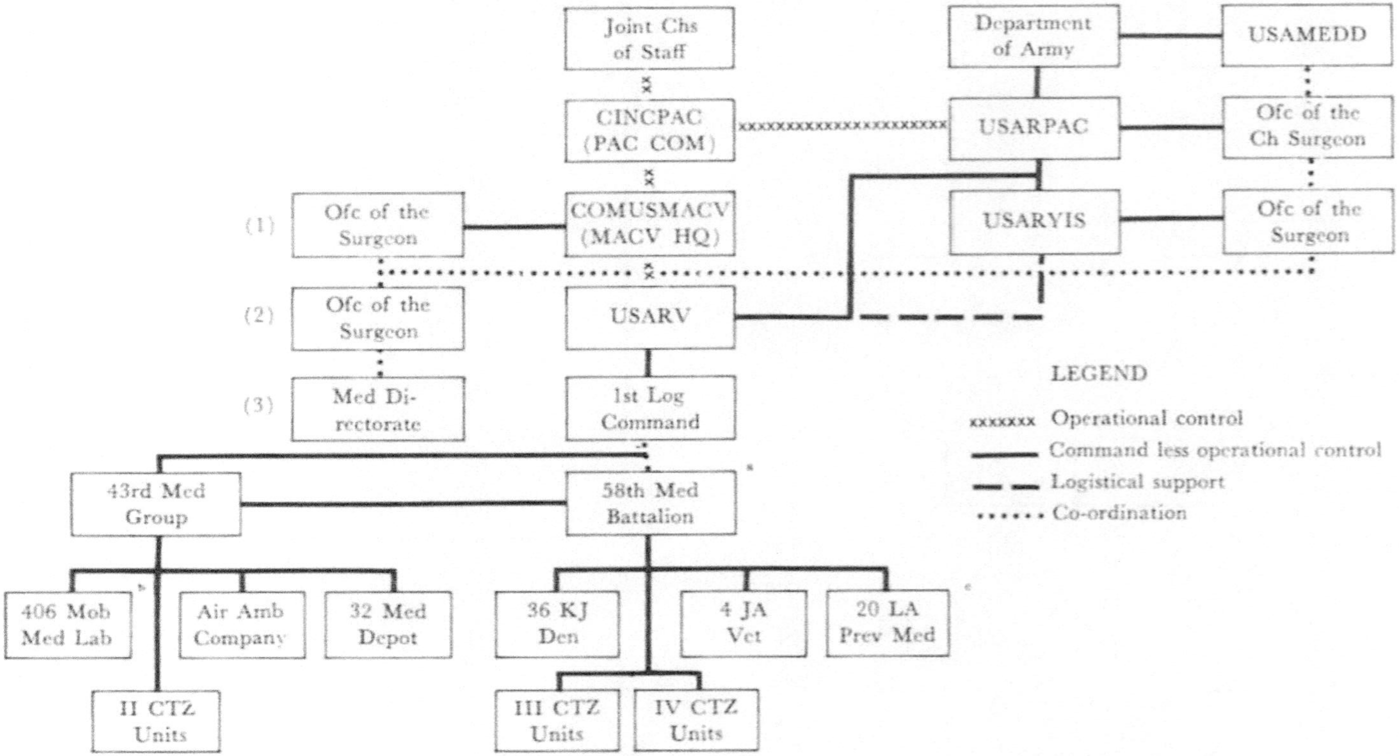

(1) Office of the Surgeon: MACV [d]

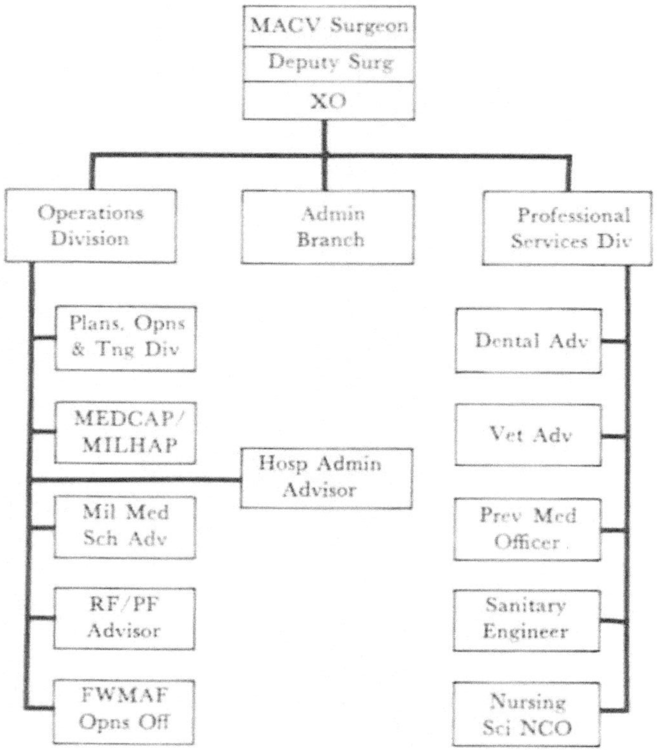

Office of the Surgeon: USARV [e] (2)

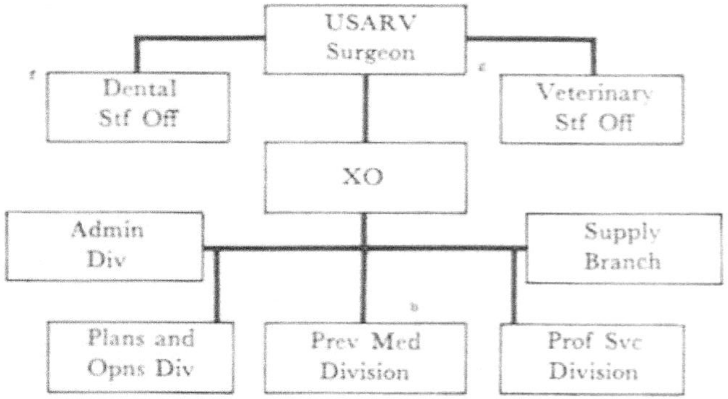

(3)

Medical Directorate: 1st Log Command [i]

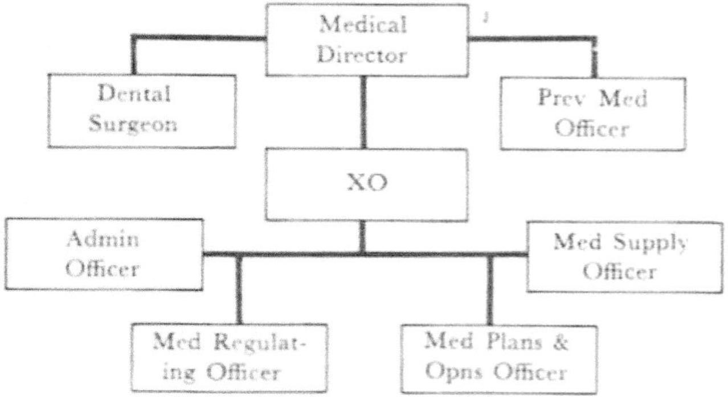

ponent headquarters rather than the commanding officer of the medical brigade.

Thus, when the advance party of the 44th Medical Brigade, activated at Fort Sam Houston, Tex., on New Year's Day 1966, arrived in Vietnam on 18 March, it was assigned to the 1st Logistical Command. A Medical Brigade (Provisional) was established, consolidating in a single element command and control responsibility for medical units not organic to divisions and separate brigades—responsibilities formerly divided between the 43d and 68th Medical Groups. As director of the

---

NOTES TO CHART 2

[a] As is indicated above, the 58th Medical Battalion, senior Army-level medical unit in Vietnam from 20 May 1965 to 31 October 1965, retained considerable command and control jurisdiction after the 43d Medical Group became operational, although it was technically a subordinate unit of that group.

[b] The 406th Mobile Medical Laboratory, based in Japan, was reorganized on 24 September 1965 to include a mobile laboratory unit attached to USASCV. Envisioned as a Pacific Command-wide laboratory service for all U.S. military medical facilities, the 406th Mobile Medical Laboratory replaced and absorbed the personnel and equipment of the 7th Medical Laboratory, previously operative in Vietnam. Throughout the Vietnam conflict, the 406th Mobile Medical Laboratory remained under the command of USARJ (United States Army, Japan). While operating in Vietnam, however, it was attached to and operationally controlled by various in-country medical headquarters.

[c] Operational control of the 36th Medical Detachment (Dental Service), 4th Medical Detachment (Veterinary Food Inspection), and 20th Preventive Medicine Unit was retained by the 1st Logistical Command Surgeon.

[d] The staff structure of the Office of the Surgeon, Headquarters, MACV, as of 31 December 1965. The consolidation of MAAGV and MACV Headquarters led to an expansion in the functions of the Office of the Surgeon, and culminated in the staff organization depicted above. The MACV Surgeon's Office changed little in subsequent years. Throughout the Vietnam conflict, Army medical staffs and headquarters were directed to co-ordinate their activities with the MACV Surgeon's Office, although the latter was not an element in the command and control chain for Army medical Units.

[e] The staff structure of the USARV Surgeon's Office as of 31 December 1965. The organizational structure was patterned after the reorganized USASCV Medical Section of 9–20 July 1965.

[f] On 1 November 1965, a full-time USARV Dental Surgeon, with no additional duties, was appointed. The commanding officer of the 36th Medical Detachment, who had previously performed that advisory function as an additional duty, continued to wear a second hat as the 1st Logistical Command Dental Surgeon.

[g] The commanding officer of the 4th Medical Detachment was also Veterinary Staff Officer in the Office of the Surgeon, USARV Headquarters, until that advisory function was delegated to lower headquarters, the 44th Medical Brigade, in 1966.

[h] Through 28 November 1965, the commanding officer of the 20th Preventive Medicine Unit served also as Preventive Medicine Officer on the staff of the USARV Surgeon. Thereafter, that position constituted a full-time assignment.

[i] The staff structure of the 1st Logistical Command Medical Directorate as of 31 December 1965. Emerging duplication in medical staff functions is reflected in the similarity between the organizations of the USARV Surgeon's Office and the Medical Directorate.

[j] Before 26 January 1966, the Medical Director was also the 1st Logistical Command Surgeon. Both were additional duties performed by the commanding officer of the 43d Medical Group, who retained his second position as 1st Logistical Command Surgeon following the appointment of a full-time Medical Director on 26 January.

Sources: (1) Medical Activities Report, Office of the Surgeon, Headquarters, Military Assistance Command, Vietnam, 1965. (2) Army Medical Service Activities Report, Office of the Surgeon, Headquarters, United States Army, Vietnam, 1965, 1966. (3) Army Medical Service Activities Report, Medical Section, Headquarters, 1st Logistical Command, 1965. (4) Army Medical Service Activities Reports, Headquarters, 43d Medical Group, 1965 and 1966. (5) Army Medical Service Activities Reports, Headquarters, 58th Medical Battalion, 1965 and 1966.

FASCOM medical section and designated commanding officer of the incoming brigade, Colonel Wier had paved the way for the assimilation of the Logistical Command's medical directorate personnel and functions into the Medical Brigade (Provisional).

The medical directorate was, at that time, charged with an inclusive mission: to develop, co-ordinate, and supervise medical plans and operations, medical supply and maintenance policies, medical statistics and records, professional medical and dental activities, preventive medicine, and medical regulating activities for all nondivisonal medical units in Vietnam. Between 18 March and 1 May, when the 44th Medical Brigade became operational, the responsibility for the accomplishment of these functions was shifted from the directorate to the brigade. The number of personnel staffing the FASCOM medical section gradually diminished; some transferred to the Medical Brigade (Provisional), others rotated. By 1 May, the only personnel left in the medical directorate were the director and a FASCOM staff medical section consisting of two plans officers, one supply and maintenance officer, one medical noncommissioned officer, and two enlisted men. Five months later, the medical section had withered even further, and was thereafter maintained at Headquarters, 1st Logistical Command, for liaison purposes only. During its 6-week span, the Medical Brigade (Provisional) had served as a medium for transferring direct command and control of medical units from the 1st Logistical Command to the 44th Medical Brigade.

From 1 May 1966 through 9 August 1967, when the most rapid buildup of U.S. combat forces took place in Vietnam, the 44th Medical Brigade remained subordinate to the 1st Logistical Command. As combat forces expanded, medical units and personnel grew proportionately; by 31 December 1966, units assigned to the medical brigade totaled 121, while assigned personnel increased from 3,187 on 1 May to 7,830 by the end of the year.

Units and individuals under the centralized control of the 44th Medical Brigade operated on a direct support/general support basis. Those providing countrywide or general support services, such as medical laboratories, supply depots, and preventive medicine units, were retained under the direct command of Headquarters, 44th Medical Brigade. Commanders of these general support facilities frequently held two posts, acting as staff officers at brigade headquarters. They were occasionally given a third hat as well, maintaining an office at USARV headquarters as staff advisers to the USARV surgeon.

Other units, particularly evacuation and treatment facilities, provided area or direct support, and as such would be subordinated to one of the medical groups. Groups were in turn assigned geographic areas of responsibility approximately equivalent to doctrinal Army corps areas, and attached to one of three area support commands of the 1st Logistical Command for administration and logistics. Thus, when the 55th Medical Group became operational in June 1966, it was attached to the Qui Nhon Area Support Command, assuming control over nondivisional medical units in II CTZ North. The 43d Medical Group, previously responsible for medical service throughout II CTZ, retained that wider responsibility only for air evacuation. For all other aspects of nondivisional medical care, the 43d Medical Group was responsible only for II CTZ South, supported in its mission by the Nha Trang (later Cam Ranh Bay) Area Support Command. Headquarters, 68th Medical Group, remained the command and control element for units in III and IV CTZ, and was, along with Headquarters, 44th Medical Brigade, and all general support units, attached to the Saigon Area Support Command for administration and logistics. (*Chart 3*)

In his assigned area, the group commander would act as the support command surgeon, providing first-echelon medical care for nondivisional and nonaviation units, plus evacuation and second-echelon medical treatment for all U.S. Army and other authorized personnel. Medical regulating within the CTZ would be controlled from his group headquarters, with all hospitalization and air ambulance units kept directly under group command. In most cases, however, a separate medical battalion headquarters would be used as the command element for ground ambulance, clearing, and dispensary units.

Had all medical command and control been vertically integrated, that system of area medical service might have been most efficient. However, the separation of administrative and logistical support from command, in conjunction with the existence of an intermediate, nonmedical headquarters between medical practitioners in the field and consultants in the USARV surgeon's office, created duplicative, overlapping, and confusing channels of communication. Administrative support was often confused with command responsibility, with actions of the former type following a communications channel from the support command directly to Headquarters, 1st Logistical Command, completely bypassing Headquarters, 44th Medical Brigade. The resultant lack of responsiveness to administrative problems on the part of the Commanding Officer, 44th Medical Brigade, an officer on the same command level as the commanding officers of each area support command, was inevitable, although difficult to explain to the Commanding General, 1st Logistical Command.

Similarly, the inability of hospital and medical group commanders to accomplish required personnel changes in their commands limited the effectiveness of medical service. Professional consultants assigned to the USARV surgeon's office, following visits to treatment facilities, made recommendations directly to the USARV surgeon or brigade personnel officer. Medical officers, on that basis, were subsequently transferred among installations and support areas, frequently without the foreknowledge of affected hospital and medical group commanders.

Duplication of Effort: Headquarters, 44th Medical Brigade, Versus the Office of the Surgeon, Headquarters, USARV

Much, if not all of that confusion, could have been eliminated through a concise delineation of the responsibilities of Headquarters, 44th Medical Brigade, vis-a-vis the USARV surgeon's office. In theory, the former should have been responsible for the day-to-day operations of all nondivisional medical services in Vietnam; the latter, for long-range plans and operations. In reality, those functions could not be so easily segregated.

In addition to those responsibilities earlier transferred from the 1st Logistical Command medical directorate to the medical brigade, the duties of the brigade commander included all in-country communications among nondivisional medical units; the evaluation and dissemination of medical intelligence; and provision for the security of all medical forces assigned to the 1st Logistical Command.

The mission of the USARV surgeon, originally less broad with respect to the operations of nondivisional medical service than that of the 1st Logistical Command surgeon, rapidly outpaced that of the commanding officer of the 44th Medical Brigade. On 10 June 1966, Colonel Wier became USARV surgeon, and command of the brigade was transferred to Colonel Ray L. Miller, MC. Exactly 5 months later, Colonel Wier received his first star. Although, when serving as brigade commander, he had expressed the desire to reduce if not eliminate the USARV surgeon's office, Brigadier General Wier found it necessary to double the size of his office staff over the next year. As U.S. Army forces and their organic medical units expanded, so, of course, did the workload of the surgeon assigned to headquarters of the Army component. However, part of the growth in the USARV surgeon's office was the result of an increasing volume of paperwork, principally planning, accomplished at the Army level. Much of that planning was demanded of General Wier by G–3, Assistant Chief of Staff for Plans and Operations, Headquarters, USARV. Because of the timelag involved, General Wier found co-ordination with Headquarters, 44th Medical Brigade, difficult and was therefore unwillingly forced to increase the staff of his plans and operations division. Other responsibilities such as collecting and compiling medical statistics were added to his office during the year, and could not be delegated to lower headquarters. Professional activities and consultants had to remain at the Army level for, in addition to visit-

CHART 3—MEDICAL COMMAND AND STAFF STRUCTURE, U.S. ARMY, VIETNAM, 1 MAY 1966–10 AUGUST 1967

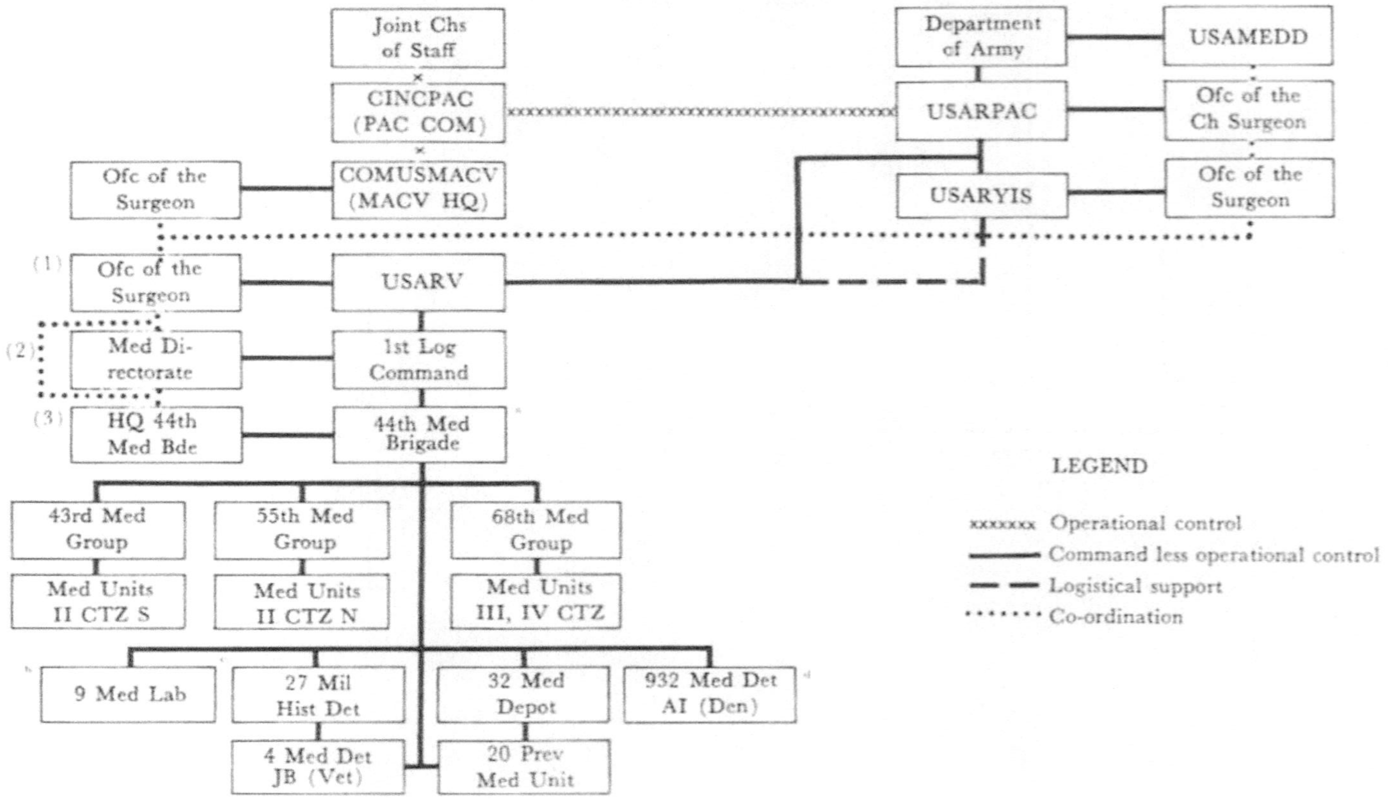

(1) Office of the Surgeon: USARV [a]

(2) Medical Directorate 1st Logistical Command [g]

(3) Headquarters 44th Medical Brigade [i]

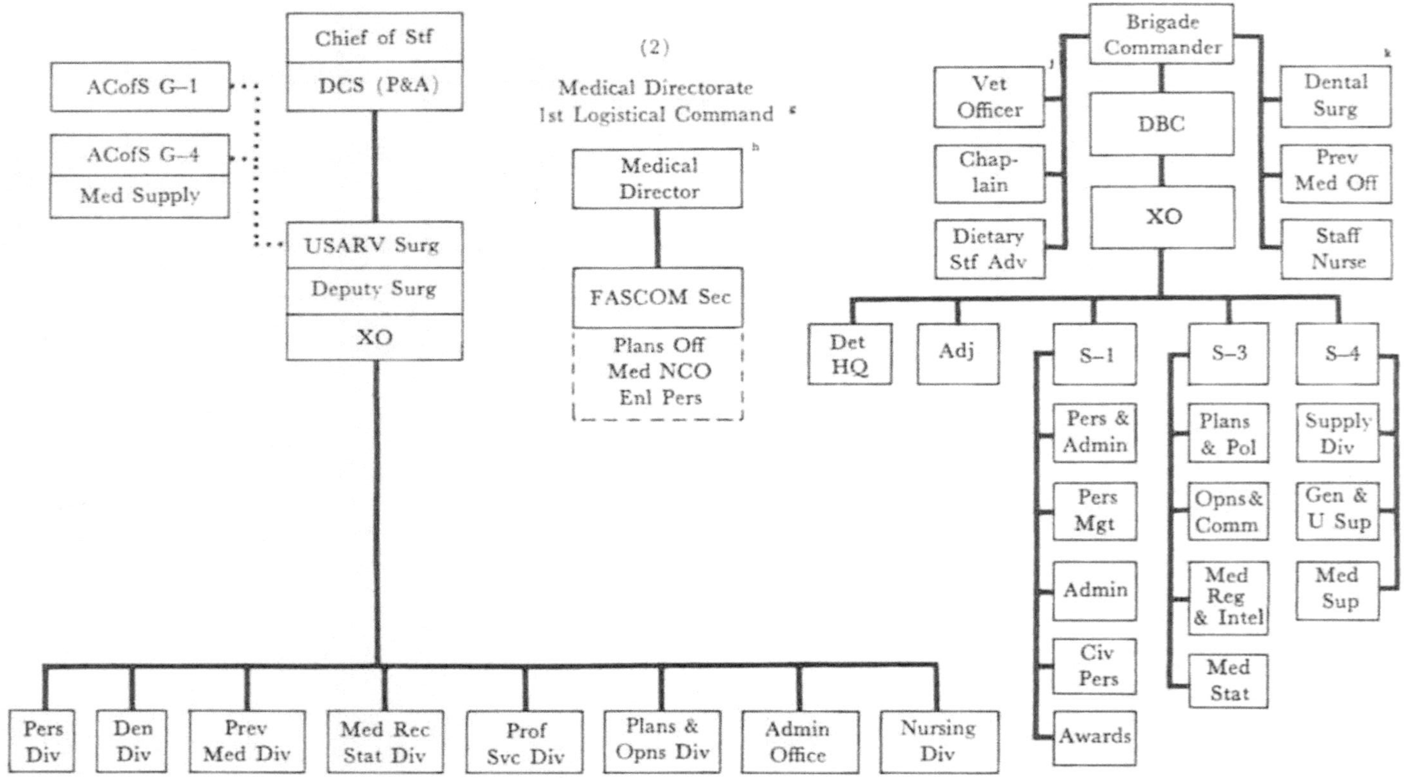

ing hospitals, they provided consultant services for organic medical units in divisions outside the purview of the 44th Medical Brigade.

The confusion in command and control, support, and co-ordination that ensued was documented in a position paper prepared by General Wier in June 1967. Noting that the USARV surgeon was not only the senior medical officer, but was also assisted by the most competent medical consultants in Vietnam, General Wier argued for the placement of the 44th Medical Brigade directly under Headquarters, USARV. To do so would make the highest level of medical skill directly and immediately available to all medical units; a level of skill far beyond that available to the Commanding General, 1st Logistical Command, under the existing organization. Advantages resulting from the removal of the medical brigade and subordinate units from the intermediate logistics headquarters would be numerous: reinforcement of the medical service of tactical units could be more rapidly effected, and personnel economies could be realized through the realignment of duplicative staffs in higher and lower medical headquarters and through the elimination of the 1st

---

NOTES TO CHART 3

[a] Deployment of medical groups as of 1 July 1966. When the 68th Medical Group became operational on 18 February 1966, it became the higher headquarters for, and assumed the former command and control responsibilities of, the 58th Medical Battalion. The 55th Medical Group became operational on 1 July 1966, assuming control over nondivisional medical units in the northern portion of II CTZ. The 43d Medical Group remained the command and control element for units in the southern portion of II CTZ. It acted in the same capacity for the 6th Convalescent Center, operational at Cam Ranh Bay since 16 May 1966, although doctrine specified that the facility be assigned directly to Headquarters, 44th Medical Brigade. All Medical Groups were further attached for administration and logistics to the headquarters of the various area support commands, subordinate commands of the 1st Logistical Command.

[b] On 1 August 1966, Headquarters, 9th Medical Laboratory became operational in Saigon. Thereafter, it acted as the control element for all medical laboratories in Vietnam, including the 406th Medical Mobile Laboratory.

[c] Attached for administration and logistics.

[d] Upon becoming operational in Saigon on 27 December 1965, the 932d Medical Detachment (AI) became the command and control element for dental units in Vietnam.

[e] The staff structure of the USARV Surgeon's Office as of 31 December 1966.

[f] Until 9 March 1967, the Chief Nurse, USARV Surgeon's Office, also acted as Staff Nurse, Headquarters, 44th Medical Brigade. From 9 March to 27 September, the latter position was occupied on a full-time basis by an ANC officer.

[g] The staff structure of the 1st Logistical Command Medical Directorate as of 1 October 1966.

[h] The primary duty of the 1st Logistical Command Medical Director was Commanding Officer, 44th Medical Brigade.

[i] The staff structure of Headquarters, 44th Medical Brigade, as of 31 December 1966. In general, the organization differed in structure from that of the Medical Brigade (Provisional) only in the addition of two officers to the Brigade Commander's staff: (1) The History Staff Advisor; and (2) the Staff Nurse.

[j] On 6 June 1966, the Brigade Staff Veterinarian was appointed to additional duty as Veterinary Consultant to the USARV Surgeon.

[k] The primary duty of the 44th Medical Brigade Dental Surgeon was commanding officer of the 932d Medical Detachment (Dental Service).

Sources: (1) Army Medical Service Activities Reports, Office of the Surgeon, Headquarters, United States Army, Vietnam, 1965, 1966, and 1967. (2) Army Medical Service Activities Report, Headquarters, 44th Medical Brigade, 1966. (3) Interview, Brigadier General James A. Wier, MC, USARV Surgeon, and Captain Darrell G. McPherson, MSC, 17 June 1967.

Logistical Command medical directorate. Perhaps most importantly, the centralized control of all Army medical assets in Vietnam would permit the most efficient use of critical, scarce resources. Their optimal utilization would be assured by vesting in the senior medical officer in Vietnam, the USARV surgeon, full command and control responsibility.

With the exception of G–1, Assistant Chief of Staff for Personnel, all members of the USARV General Staff concurred in General Wier's proposal. The lone demurral argued that placing the medical brigade directly under USARV headquarters would cause the latter to become a support command, rather than the command and control headquarters for a true field army. General Wier's paper was returned without action, and before the proposal could be resubmitted, he returned to the United States, replaced as USARV surgeon by Brigadier General (later Major General) Glenn J. Collins, MC.

The effort to elevate the 44th Medical Brigade to the field-army level of command did not subside, and events of the first 2 weeks of General Collins' tour as USARV surgeon were to conspire to make that effort successful. As the result of decisions made elsewhere, space ceilings were placed on USARV in July 1967, bringing about a total reevaluation of the Army medical service in Vietnam. After a careful examination of the over-all Army medical support structure, the Office of the Surgeon concluded that spaces could be deleted from the division medical service. To do so, however, would make it mandatory that the USARV surgeon have complete and direct control over all medical resources. Otherwise, the immediate reinforcement of divisional medical units could not be guaranteed.

On 2 August 1967, a final realignment study including these qualifications was presented by General Collins to the USARV General Staff. More explicit than the June proposal, it listed in detail both the advantages of assigning the 44th Medical Brigade directly to USARV, as well as the disadvantages of leaving the brigade directly under the 1st Logistical Command. Two points were, for the first time, emphasized: the reduction in delays in medical planning and medical statistical reporting, and in implementing the recommendations of professional consultants; and the greater ease in the management of medical personnel to be realized by assigning the brigade directly to USARV headquarters.

Nondivisional Command and Staff Relationships: 1967–71

The need could no longer be denied. On 10 August 1967, the 44th Medical Brigade was released from the 1st Logistical Command and reassigned directly to USARV as a major subordinate unit. (*Chart 4*) The efforts of the last 2 years were rewarded; the arguments of

Chart 4—Medical Command and Staff Structure, U.S. Army, Vietnam, 10 August 1967–1 March 1970

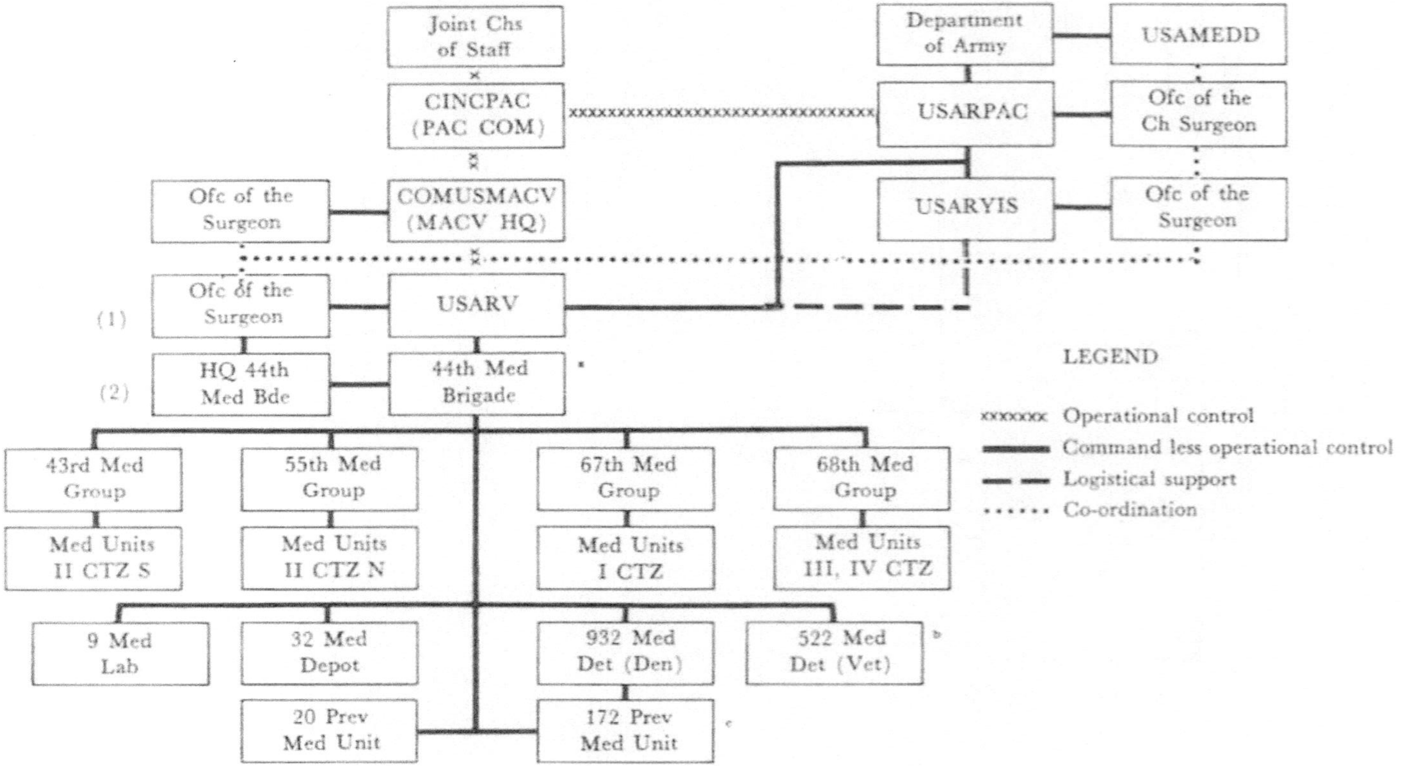

(1) Office of the Surgeon: USARV [d]

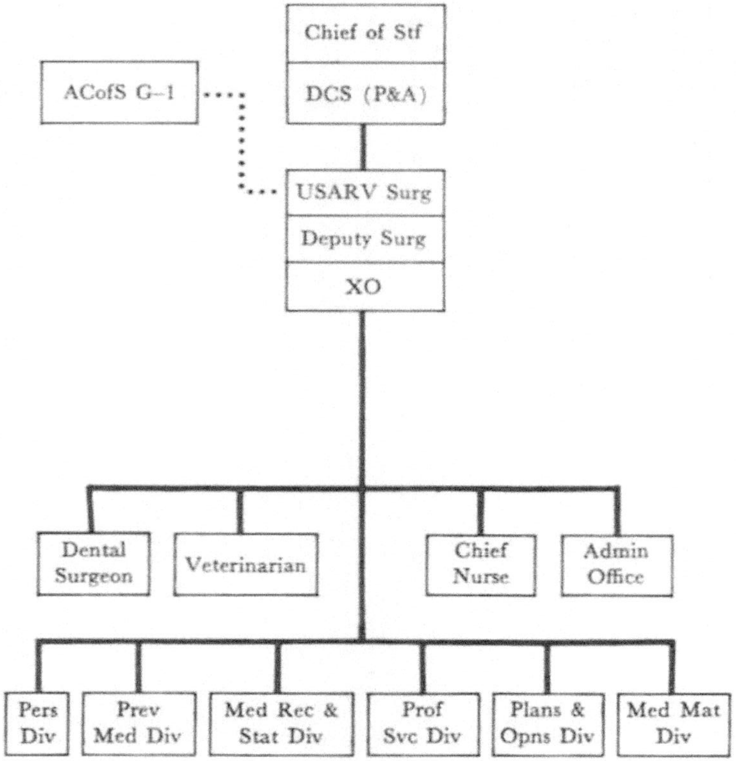

(2) Headquarters 44th Medical Brigade [e]

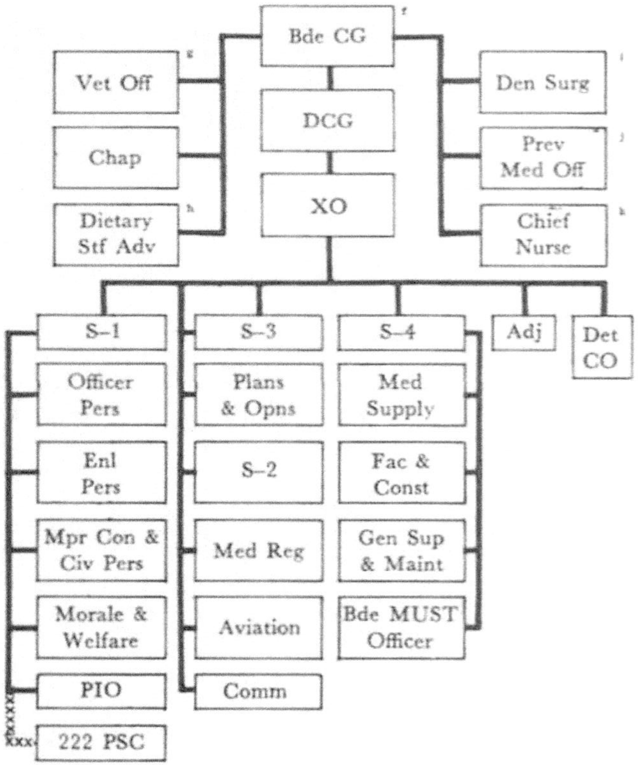

General Heaton, General Steger, General Wier, General Collins, and Colonel Neel, validated. The Army medical service in Vietnam became in effect what it would become in later years in name—a unified medical command.

The Medical Brigade as a Major Subordinate Command of USARV Headquarters

General Collins assumed the dual role of Surgeon, USARV, and Commanding General, 44th Medical Brigade. Although technically excluded in the former capacity from operational control over nondivisional medical units, he was nonetheless able to exercise full command and control responsibilities in his other position as brigade commander.

As USARV surgeon, General Collins and his staff were charged with five general responsibilities: to advise the USARV commander on all matters regarding the health of the command; exercise technical supervision over all medical activities of the command; plan to assure the availability of adequate medical support in the command; control the assignment and use of medical personnel in Vietnam; and manage medical supply and maintenance functions. As applied to nondivisional medical service, these were interpreted as responsibilities for medium- and long-range planning, the development of theater-wide medical planning factors, and the monitoring of co-ordination between the 44th Medical Brigade and supported units.

Meanwhile, Headquarters, 44th Medical Brigade, assumed responsibility for programs not originally envisioned for a field medical unit, in-

---

NOTES TO CHART 4

[a] The maximum deployment of medical groups in Vietnam, a situation existing from 22 October 1967, when the 67th Medical Group became operational, to the 15 June 1969 deactivation of the 55th Medical Group. Originally headquartered in III CTZ, the 67th Medical Group relocated in I CTZ early in 1968.

[b] The 522d Medical Detachment (AF) became operational on 10 April 1968, assuming control over all veterinary TOE units in Vietnam.

[c] The 172d Preventive Medicine Unit became operational under reduced strength on 1 August 1968. It was not subordinated to the 20th Preventive Medicine Unit, but rather assigned directly to Headquarters, 44th Medical Brigade. Both the 172d and 20th Preventive Medicine Units acted as control elements for preventive medicine detachments in Vietnam, the former for those operative in I and II N CTZ, the latter for units in II S, III, and IV CTZ.

[d] The staff structure of the USARV Surgeon's Office as of 31 December 1969.

[e] The staff structure of Headquarters, 44th Medical Brigade as of 31 December 1968.

[f] The Commanding General of the 44th Medical Brigade was also USARV Surgeon.

[g] The 44th Medical Brigade Veterinary Officer was also USARV Veterinarian.

[h] The 44th Medical Brigade Dietary Staff Adviser performed additional duty as Dietetic Consultant in the USARV Surgeon's Office.

[i] The 44th Medical Brigade Dental Surgeon was also USARV Dental Surgeon.

[j] The 44th Medical Brigade Preventive Medicine Officer was also USARV Preventive Medicine Officer.

[k] The 44th Medical Brigade Chief Nurse was also Chief Nurse, USARV Surgeon's Office.

Sources: (1) Army Medical Service Activities Reports, Office of the Surgeon, Headquarters, United States Army, Vietnam, 1965, 1967, and 1969. (2) Army Medical Service Activities Report, Headquarters, 44th Medical Brigade, 1968.

cluding an awards program, command maintenance inspections, and supervision of special services activities. Other responsibilities of the brigade commander and his staff were more limited than those of the USARV surgeon, including in-country medical regulating and the short-term planning of day-to-day operations involving army level medical support.

The similarity in functions performed by these two medical staffs produced both advantages and disadvantages. Personnel economies were realized, and the degree of co-ordination between higher and lower headquarters enhanced, but considerable confusion remained as to the precise staff functions to be performed at each level, especially with respect to operational responsibilites.

In addition to the surgeon/brigade commander, the dental surgeon, chief nurse, veterinary officer, preventive medicine officer, entomologist, dietitian, and aviation staff officer sat on both staffs, eliminating several duplicate slots. Further, personnel consultants on the USARV surgeon's staff now had direct access to medical treatment facilities of the brigade, contributing to improved relations between surgeons and medical commanders at all levels. The greater ease of co-ordination which these staffing arrangements permitted was heightened by the shift in location of brigade headquarters from Tan Son Nhut to Long Binh late in September 1967. The proximity of the two headquarters added materially to the freedom of communications between the two staffs. As General Neel, successor to General Collins as USARV surgeon/brigade commander, emphasized, good communications were essential to the success of army level medical service in Vietnam.

All forms of co-ordination between the two staffs were not enhanced by the assignment of the medical brigade directly to USARV headquarters, however. In an attempt to delineate the proper role of S-3, Plans and Operations, the USARV Organization and Functions Manual was amended in December 1968, and the name of the USARV surgeon's Plans and Operations Division changed to the Plans, Programs, and Analysis Division. That abortive attempt to more precisely describe the division's functions created more confusion than order, and it reverted to the originai designation the following year. In short, under the existing medical structure in Vietnam, no better description of proper staff functions could be made on the simple statement: the brigade staff were the operators; the surgeon's staff, the advisers and long-range planners.

Establishment of the U.S. Army Medical Command, Vietnam

Duplicative staff functions, the last major area of deficiency in the medical command and control structure in Vietnam, were eliminated in 1970 with the creation of USAMEDCOMV (U.S. Army Medical Command, Vietnam) (Provisional). The previous year had been one of major reorganization, consolidation, and realignment of 44th Medical Brigade units. Headquarters, 55th Medical Group, had been deactivated on 15 June. The 43d Medical Group then assumed command and control over all 55th Medical Group units in II CTZ, but was itself scheduled for deactivation in the spring of 1970. When Headquarters, 43d Medical Group, was reduced to zero strength, the 67th Medical Group, which had become operational in October 1967 and had assumed command and control over nondivisonal units in I CTZ, became the command and control element for medical units in II CTZ as well. Throughout, the 68th Medical Group exercised responsibility for nondivisional medical service in III and IV CTZ.

Reorganization and consolidation of medical staffs proceeded in tandem with that of field units. A review of functions performed by the USARV surgeon's office and the 44th Medical Brigade headquarters suggested that, if the two staffs were combined, duplication and overlap could be eliminated. Accordingly, Brigadier General David E. Thomas, MC, USARV surgeon/brigade commander, appointed a study group to determine the feasibility of such a move. A lone admonition guided their study: that the prospective consolidation of staffs and functions result in no loss in the efficiency of medical service in Vietnam.

A basic organization and function for the unified medical command was derived from the finding of the study group. The 44th Medical Brigade would be eliminated, with all command and control responsibilities absorbed by the medical command. The USARV surgeon would assume the role of Commanding General, USAMEDCOMV. Similarly, the Deputy Commander, USAMEDCOMV, would serve as the USARV deputy surgeon. Manpower spaces would be eliminated in the offices of the USAMEDCOMV dental surgeon and veterinarian, officers who had formerly maintained staffs in both medical headquarters. In total, the study revealed that manpower could be reduced by 17 percent with no loss in functional efficiency through the proposed consolidation of medical staffs. Based on these projected results, the study further recommended that, in the future, the dual function concept of the surgeon as commander of the major surbordinate medical unit be retained, and considered on all levels as a method of reducing manpower requirements and achieving the best utilization of all scarce medical resources.

On 1 March 1970, Headquarters, 44th Medical Brigade, was consolidated with the USARV surgeon's office, forming the USAMEDCOMV (Provisional). (*Chart 5*) That command continues to provide field-army-level medical service throughout Vietnam. Most of the co-ordination and logistics problems associated with the Army medical structure in Vietnam have been eliminated, and benefits have been achieved through a

CHART 5—MEDICAL COMMAND AND STAFF STRUCTURE, U.S. ARMY, VIETNAM, 1 MARCH 1970

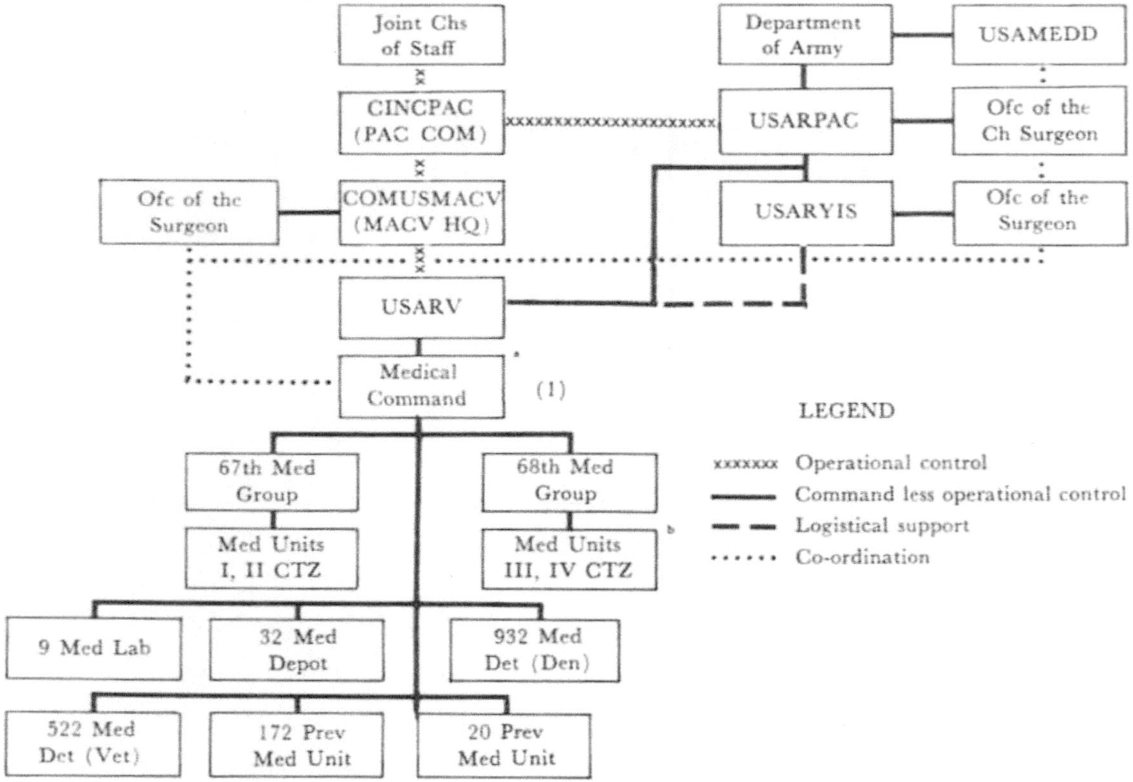

(1) Headquarters Medical Command (Provisional) [c]

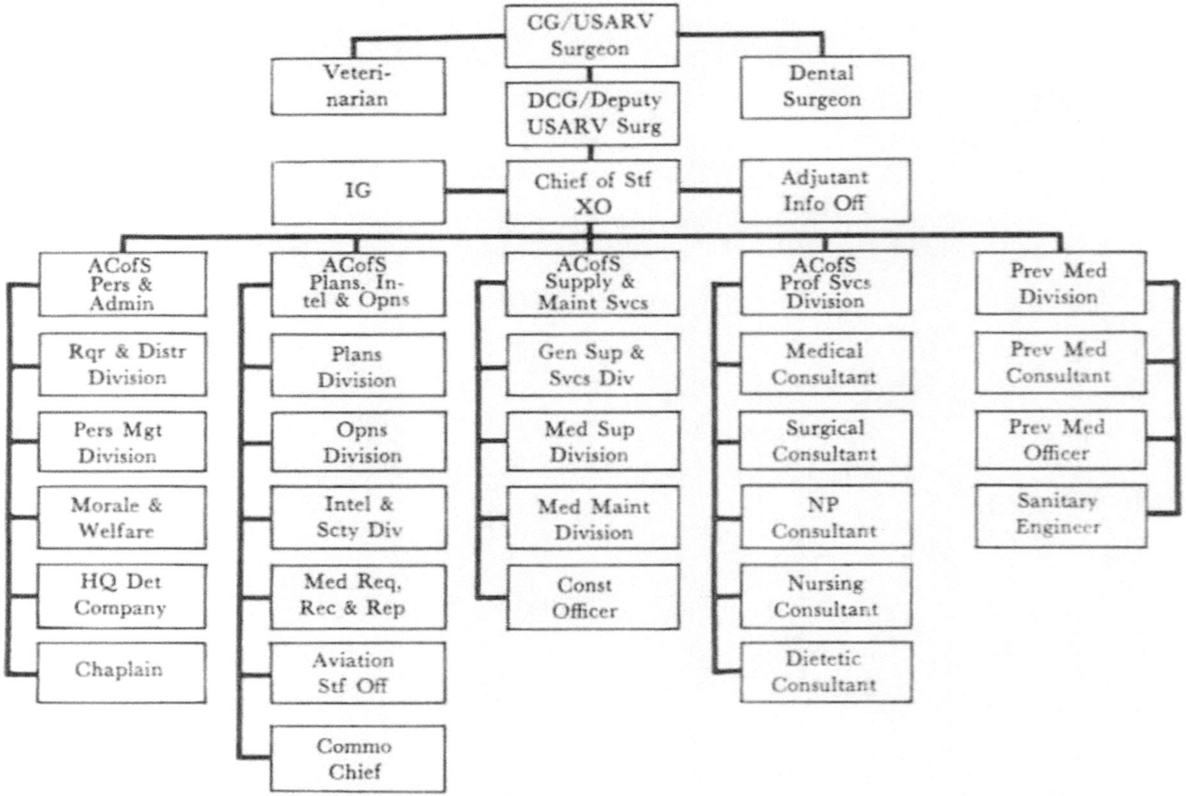

reorganization that has resulted in a medical command structure curiously similar to that which prevailed before the buildup of U.S. combat forces. Duplication of efforts in the functional areas of command, including dental and veterinary control, administration, and plans and operations, has been eliminated. Manpower requirements have been reduced without degrading the efficiency of medical operations. More importantly, the responsiveness and flexibility of the command to changes in medical support requirements have improved, perhaps the ultimate test of the value of Army medical service in the theater of operations.

NOTES TO CHART 5

[a] The deployment of Medical Groups in Vietnam has continued despite the reduction of zero personnel strength and equipment status of the 43d Medical Group on 7 February 1970.

[b] Support areas in Vietnam are now referred to as Military Regions (MR) rather than Corps Tactical Zones (CTZ). The geographic regions thus specified are similar to, although not identical with, the CTZ's of earlier years.

[c] The staff structure of Headquarters, Medical Command (Provisional) as of 1 March 1970.

Sources: (1) Army Medical Service Activities Reports, Office of the Surgeon, Headquarters, United States Army, Vietnam, 1965 and 1969. (2) Operational Report, Lessons Learned of the United States Army Medical Command, Vietnam (Provisional) for Period Ending 30 April 1970, Headquarters, United States Army Medical Command, Vietnam (Provisional), 15 May 1970.

CHAPTER II

Health of the Command

Rates and Trends

In Vietnam, as in Korea and in the Asiatic and Pacific theaters in World War II, the cumulative effect of disease was the greatest drain on the strength of the American combat and support effort. Disease admissions accounted for just over two of every three (69 percent) hospital admissions in Vietnam in the period 1965–69; battle injuries and wounds, in contrast, were responsible for approximately one of six admissions during this period. (*Table 1*) But the average hospital stay and thus the time lost from duty resulting from combat injury was considerably longer than that resulting from disease. In 1970, however, as a result of the diminution of the American combat role, disease and nonbattle injury accounted for more than half the man-days lost to the Army in that theater. (*Table 2*)

While indicative of the theater's single greatest cause of morbidity, disease rates for Vietnam revealed encouraging trends when compared to rates for previous conflicts. The average annual disease admission rate for Vietnam (351 per 1,000 per year) was approximately one-third of that for the China-Burma-India and Southwest Pacific theaters in World War II (844 per 1,000 per year and 890 per 1,000 per year, respectively), and more than 40 percent less than the rate for the Korean War (611 per 1,000 per year). (*See Table 1.*)*

One of the most striking achievements of military medicine in Vietnam was the rapid and effective establishment of a preventive medicine program that blunted the impact of disease on combat operations. In World War II, preventive medicine programs in the Far East did not begin to make inroads upon disease incidence until 1945, a year of transition from war to peace. In Korea the delay was less, but still considerable. In Vietnam, however, effective disease control programs were introduced in 1965, and these were successfully maintained throughout the stress of the troop buildup. (*See Table 1.*)

In addition to minimizing the incidence of disease in American troops, the medical effort in Vietnam had the ancillary benefit in the late 1960's

---

*Rates are expressed as cases per annum per 1,000 average strength, throughout this chapter.

TABLE 1.—HOSPITAL ADMISSIONS FOR ALL CAUSES, U.S. ARMY, IN THREE WARS: WORLD WAR II, KOREA, AND VIETNAM, BY YEAR

[Rate expressed as number of admissions per annum per 1,000 average strength]

War	Year	All causes	Non-battle injury	Battle injury and wounds	Dis-ease	Disease as percent of all causes
World War II						
China-Burma-India	1942	1,130	81	3	1,046	92
	1943	1,081	84	6	991	92
	1944	1,191	96	18	1,077	90
	1945	745	80	4	661	90
Southwest Pacific	1942	1,035	178	25	832	80
	1943	1,229	171	12	1,046	84
	1944	1,013	139	34	840	83
	1945	990	99	48	843	85
Korea	[1] 1950	1,526	242	460	824	61
	1951	897	151	170	576	64
	1952	592	102	57	433	75
Vietnam	1965	484	67	62	355	73
	1966	547	76	75	396	72
	1967	515	69	84	362	70
	1968	523	70	120	333	64
	1969	459	63	87	309	67

[1] July–December only.

Sources: (1) World War II: Morbidity and Mortality in the United States Army, 1940–1945. Preliminary Tables Based on Periodic Summary Reports, Office of the Surgeon General, U.S. Army. (2) Korea: Korea, A Summary of Medical Experience, July 1950–December 1952. Reprinted from Health of the Army, January, February, and March 1953, Office of the Surgeon General, U.S. Army. (3) Vietnam: Health of the Army, May 1966, May 1967, May 1968, May 1969, May 1970, Office of the Surgeon General, U.S. Army.

of making predictable the parameters of various disease problems at particular points in time. The curves depicting the monthly rates per 1,000 per year of those diseases having greatest impact on military operations reveal that, as the Medical Department effort became established and routinized, the annual rates fell, month by month, very closely together. Thus, the 1968 and 1969 curves for malaria, for example, were almost superimposed upon each other. (*Chart 6*) Not only was disease being controlled but, if preventive measures were properly implemented, its incidence could be forecast with increasing accuracy, and it therefore became a variable for which the field commander could account in planning combat operations.

TABLE 2.—APPROXIMATE NUMBER OF MAN-DAYS LOST FROM DUTY, BY CAUSE, AMONG U.S. ARMY PERSONNEL IN VIETNAM, 1967–70

[Preliminary estimates based on sample tabulations of individual medical records]

Cause	1967	1968	1969	1970
Malaria	228, 100	215, 400	183, 050	167, 950
Acute respiratory infection	66, 800	83, 181	63, 530	70, 800
Skin diseases (including dermatophytosis)	66, 400	64, 832	50, 790	80, 140
Neuropsychiatric conditions	70, 100	106, 743	125, 280	175, 510
Viral hepatitis	80, 700	116, 981	86, 460	85, 840
Diarrheal diseases	55, 500	60, 132	48, 980	45, 100
Venereal disease (excluding CRO [1] cases)	7, 500	6, 840	3, 130	3, 700
Fever of undetermined origin	205, 700	289, 700	201, 500	205, 500
Disease total	780, 800	943, 809	762, 720	834, 540
Battle injury and wounds	1, 505, 200	2, 522, 820	1, 992, 580	1, 044, 750
Other injury	347, 100	415, 140	374, 030	309, 670

[1] CRO: Carded for record only.

Source: Health of the Command, report submitted to the Deputy Surgeon General, March 1971.

Concentration upon prevention did not preclude the aggressive development of new treatment regimens for old and known problems. In 1965, the average time lost from duty for a patient ill with *Plasmodium vivax* malaria was 21 days, and for the *Plasmodium falciparum* malaria patient, 5 weeks. By 1969, *P. vivax* patients were being returned to duty in 5 to 8 days, and *P. falciparum* patients in 17 to 19 days. Similarly, in 1966, average time lost from duty for the patient with infectious hepatitis was 49 days; in 1970, it was 35 days.

Diseases of major military import for which the incidence in Vietnam exceeded the incidence in the Army as a whole include malaria, viral hepatitis, diarrheal diseases, diseases of the skin, FUO (fever of undetermined origin), and venereal disease. Venereal disease in Vietnam was most often gonorrhea or other infections of the urinary canal reported under this rubric on clinical grounds alone. It was treated on an outpatient basis and was not a major cause of lost duty time.

The other diseases can be divided into two rather general groups: those, such as hepatitis, which affected relatively few men but incapacitated them for long periods; and those, like most diarrheal and skin diseases endemic to Vietnam, which incapacitated large numbers of men,

CHART 6—ADMISSIONS, BY YEAR, TO HOSPITAL AND QUARTERS FOR MALARIA IN THREE WARS: WORLD WAR II, KOREA, AND VIETNAM

[Rate expressed as number of admissions per annum per 1,000 average strength]

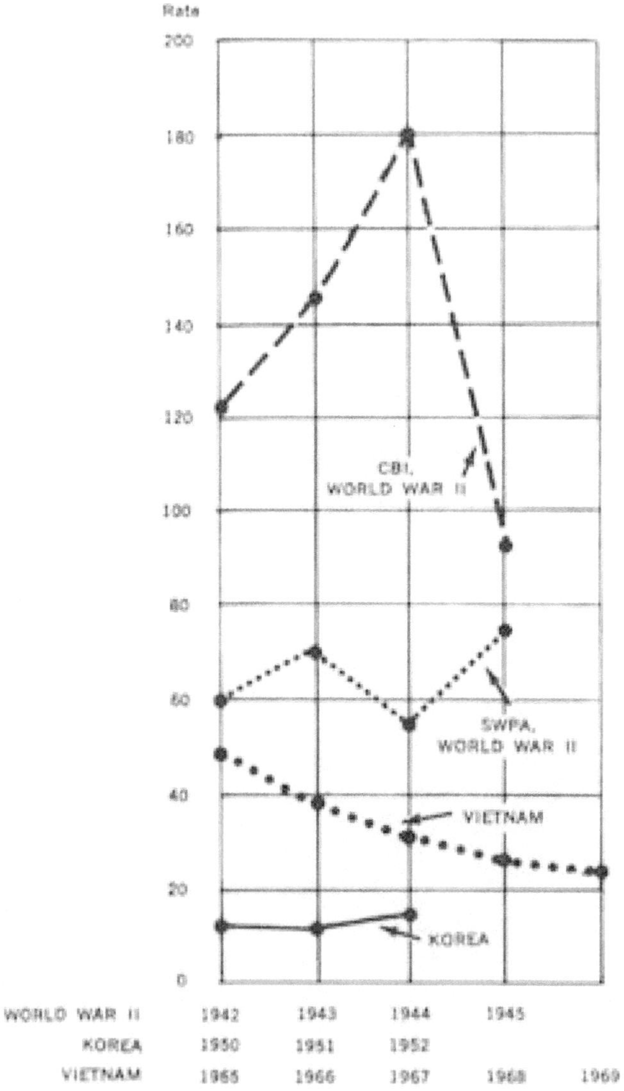

Sources: (1) World War II: Medical Department, United States Army. Preventive Medicine in World War II, Volume IV. Communicable Diseases Transmitted Chiefly Through the Respiratory and Alimentary Tracts. Washington: U.S. Government Printing Office, 1958. (2) Korea: Korea, A Summary of Medical Experience, July 1950–December 1952. Reprinted from Health of the Army, January, February, and March 1953. Office of the Surgeon General, United States Army. (3) Vietnam: Health of the Army, May 1966, May 1967, May 1968, May 1969, and May 1970. Office of the Surgeon General, United States Army.

but for relatively short periods. Malaria, and especially the drug-resistant *P. falciparum* strain, widespread and incapacitating for relatively long periods, combined the least desirable features of each of these categories and was consequently the greatest medicomilitary disease problem in Vietnam. (*Table 3*)

TABLE 3.—SELECTED CAUSES OF ADMISSIONS TO HOSPITAL AND QUARTERS AMONG ACTIVE-DUTY U.S. ARMY PERSONNEL IN VIETNAM, 1965–70

[Rate expressed as number of admissions per annum per 1,000 average strength]

Cause	1965	1966	1967	1968	1969	1970
Wounded in action	61. 6	74. 8	84. 1	120. 4	87. 6	52. 9
Injury (except wounded in action)	67. 2	75. 7	69. 1	70. 0	63. 9	59. 9
Malaria	48. 5	39. 0	30. 7	24. 7	20. 8	22. 1
Acute respiratory infections	47. 1	32. 5	33. 4	34. 0	31. 0	38. 8
Skin diseases (includes dermatophytosis)	33. 1	28. 4	28. 3	23. 2	18. 9	32. 9
Neuropsychiatric conditions	11. 7	12. 3	10. 5	13. 3	15. 8	25. 1
Viral hepatitis	5. 7	4. 0	7. 0	8. 6	6. 4	7. 2
Venereal disease (includes CRO [1])	277. 4	281. 5	240. 5	195. 8	199. 5	222. 9
Venereal disease (excludes CRO [1])	3. 6	3. 8	2. 6	2. 2	1. 0	1. 4
Fever of undetermined origin	42. 8	57. 2	56. 2	56. 7	57. 7	72. 3

[1] CRO: Carded for record only.

Source: Health of the Army, May 1966, May 1967, May 1968, May 1969, May 1970, Office of the Surgeon General, U.S. Army.

Other diseases were of grave concern to the Medical Department because of their widespread presence in the civilian population with the concomitant threat to American troops or because of their relatively exotic nature. In the first of these categories fell such conditions as plague, tuberculosis, cholera, and rabies. In the second were found such disease problems as melioidosis, Japanese B encephalitis, and amebiasis. These diseases, although constantly monitored for preventive purposes, had no material effect on U.S. fighting strength.

Statistics on hospital admissions are not an accurate guide to the extent of high-incidence, short-duration diseases, for often these conditions were treated on an outpatient basis. In 1968, for example, the Ninth Infantry Division surgeon reported that, after 5 days in the rice paddies of the Mekong Delta region, a battalion's strength was at one time reduced as much as a third by skin disease; though not fully fit for duty, most of these men were treated as outpatients. Similarly, statistics on diarrheal disease are commonly considered to reflect a small but unknown fraction of noneffectiveness caused by that problem.

A parallel problem is posed by FUO because of the tendency in the field to report such miscellaneous nonfebrile conditions as headache and backache within this category. One informed observer contends that between one-quarter and one-third of the disease reported as FUO was not in fact febrile illness. Statistics on malaria and infectious hepatitis are firmer because of the more precise nature of the categories and because of the long-term impact of the disease upon the individual patient, although studies reveal that some malaria has been reported as FUO.

Experience showed that the acclimatization process had a significant effect on the impact of the high-incidence, short-duration disease problems in Vietnam. Speaking at the 1970 Pacific Command Conference on War Surgery, Brigadier General George J. Hayes, MC, stated:

> . . . [t]here is a time reference with respect to diarrheal and upper respiratory disease and fevers of unknown origin. . . . The combination of change in circadian rhythm, climate, and early acquired diarrhea, most certainly of viral origin, lead to about a six week acclimatization period for the troops. After this time the incidence of such disorders in acclimatized troops decreases to a negligible level.

Because of the 12-month rotation policy, unacclimatized troops continually arriving in Vietnam tended to keep the rates for these diseases high.

Acclimatization was not only a physical problem but a psychological and cultural one as well, as indicated by the substantial rates of neuropsychiatric ineffectiveness in the theater, especially during the latter part of the 1965–70 period. Not all replacements, upon entering Vietnam and being assigned to a unit, were able to negotiate the period of psychological adjustment successfully, despite the salutary effect of the 1-year rotation policy. In addition, for the individual soldier, adjustment to the Vietnam environment also involved coming to grips with the use of illicit drugs among his peers. The extent of this problem, the result of which is partially reflected in rising neuropsychiatric rates, is only now being explored.

Major Problems

Malaria.

In Vietnam, the average annual rate of admission to hospital and quarters for malaria (26.7 per 1,000 per year) was about one-third of that for the Southwest Pacific theater (70.3 per 1,000 per year) and one-quarter of that for the China-Burma-India theater (101 per 1,000 per year) in World War II. (*See Chart 6, Table 1.*) Vietnam rates, however, were higher than those for the Korean War (11.2 per 1,000 per year), principally because *P. falciparum* malaria was encountered infrequently during 1950–53, and because primaquine, having just been introduced into general use, had not yet induced the development of a drug-resistant strain of the parasite.

Over-all rates do not reflect the crippling effect of malaria on American strength at the outset of the Vietnam effort. In December 1965, the over-all Army rate in Vietnam reached a peak of 98.4 per 1,000 per year; during that period, rates for certain units operating in the Ia Drang valley were as high as 600 per 1,000 per year, and at least two maneuver battalions were rendered ineffective by malaria.

Malaria rates among military personnel in Vietnam were cyclical, reaching their low in February or March and their high in October or November. Rates correlate with climatic conditions, region of operation, and degree of contact with the enemy. (*Chart 7*) Studies done from 1965 to mid-1967 showed that, in the central highlands, enemy soldiers provided a reservoir for infection by the malaria parasite, especially the *P. falciparum* strain.

The progressive gains of the antimalaria program can be measured by the difference between the peak and bottom monthly rates in each year of the American presence. The smaller the difference, the more effective the program has been in curbing malaria. In 1965, the differ-

CHART 7—ADMISSIONS TO HOSPITAL AND QUARTERS FOR MALARIA AMONG U.S. ARMY PERSONNEL IN VIETNAM, 1965–69

[Rate expressed as number of admissions per annum per 1,000 average strength]

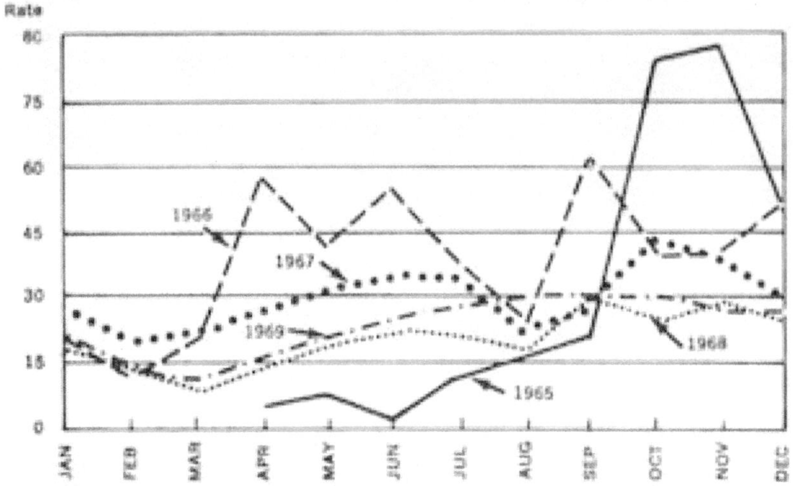

Source: Health of the Army, May 1966, May 1967, May 1968, May 1969, and May 1970. Office of the Surgeon General, United States Army.

ence between these two rates was 97.1; in 1969, it was 20.7. Success was also indicated by the down trend, since 1967, in the absolute number of malaria cases, and by the low level at which deaths from malaria have been held:

Year	*Cases*	*Deaths*
1965	1,972	16
1966	6,662	14
1967	9,124	11
1968	8,616	15
1969	7,322	10
1970	6,718	12

Much of the success in the fight against malaria was the result of the ongoing preventive medicine program and of findings of Army researchers in the field and the laboratory. Advances also were made in the treatment of the disease once it had been incurred, advances which lowered the relapse rate and returned the soldier to duty more quickly.

In mid-1966, a multiple treatment regimen consisting of quinine, pyrimethamine, and dapsone was instituted for the initial attack of *P. falciparum*. Before the addition of dapsone to this regimen, relapse rates averaged 7 to 8 percent; after the change, they were lowered to 2 to 3 percent. Studies done in 1969 and 1970 at the 6th Convalescent Center, however, indicated that, among patients who received this regimen orally, the relapse rate had increased to about 10 percent. For those re-treated with quinine orally, the relapse rate was 67 percent; with intravenous quinine, 11 percent. These observations suggest that the *P. falciparum* malaria parasite acquires substantial resistance to quinine, a phenomenon that demands further study.

Plasmodium vivax malaria was experienced very rarely in American troops until mid-1967. Since then, largely because of breakdowns in malaria discipline, it has become an increasingly large factor in the problem with this disease in Vietnam. *P. vivax* infection has been easily treated with a short course of chloroquine followed by primaquine. A further problem with this strain, however, arose with its increasing appearance in the United States in Vietnam returnees, an experience which paralleled that of the American forces in Korea.

In 1965, 62 cases of malaria were treated in Army facilities in the United States. In 1970, 2,222 such cases were treated, and this figure is a minimum, neglecting cases that arose in returnees after separation from the service. Eighty percent of these stateside cases of malaria were of the *P. vivax* variety. This graphically pointed to a failure in the terminal prophylaxis program, which, as a result, has received further command emphasis during 1970:

Year	*Cases*
1965	62
1966	303
1967	2, 021
1968	1, 598
1969	1, 969
1970	2, 222

Hepatitis

As with malaria, the average annual infectious hepatitis rate in Vietnam (6.9 per 1,000 per year) was lower than comparable rates for World War II (SWPA, 27.1 per 1,000 per year; CBI, 9.8 per 1,000 per year), but unlike malaria, Vietnam rates for infectious hepatitis were also lower than those for Korea (7.9 per 1,000 per year). (*See Table 1; Chart 8*). The hepatitis rate in Vietnam reached a peak in August 1968;

CHART 8—ADMISSIONS, BY YEAR, TO HOSPITAL AND QUARTERS FOR HEPATITIS IN THREE WARS: WORLD WAR II, KOREA, AND VIETNAM

[Rate expressed as number of admissions per annum per 1,000 average strength]

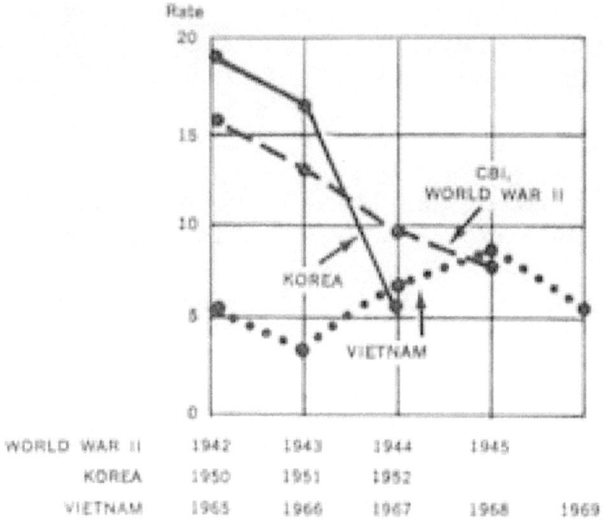

Sources: (1) World War II: Medical Department, United States Army. Preventive Medicine in World War II. Volume IV. Communicable Diseases Transmitted Chiefly Through Respiratory and Alimentary Tracts. Washington: U.S. Government Printing Office, 1958. (2) Korea: Korea. A Summary of Medical Experience, July 1950–December 1952. Reprinted from Health of the Army, January, February, and March 1953. Office of the Surgeon General, United States Army. (3) Vietnam: Health of the Army. May 1966, May 1967, May 1968, May 1969, and May 1970. Office of the Surgeon General, United States Army.

CHART 9—ADMISSIONS TO HOSPITAL AND QUARTERS FOR HEPATITIS AMONG U.S. ARMY PERSONNEL IN VIETNAM, 1965–69

[Rate expressed as number of admissions per annum per 1,000 average strength]

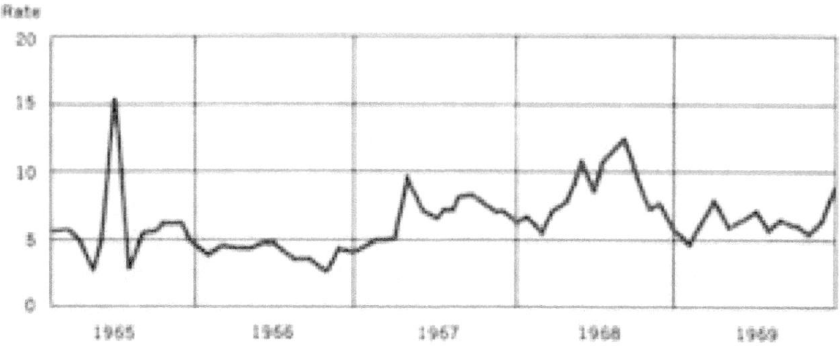

Source: Health of the Army, May 1966, May 1967, May 1968, May 1969, and May 1970, Office of the Surgeon General, United States Army.

the low rate for the theater, achieved in July 1965, has not been approached since that time. (*Chart 9*) Unlike statistics for most other disease entities in Vietnam, hepatitis incidence has not shown a downward and stabilizing trend over a period of time. Largely caused by failures in mess and field sanitation and by consumption of nonpotable water and ice available through the local economy, this disease was most commonly acquired by soldiers in their fourth through ninth month in Vietnam. The incidence of hepatitis co-varied with the occurrence of combat operations and with the degree of troop interaction with the civilian populace. Although no specific treatment was available, most patients recovered completely from viral hepatitis with adequate rest and diet. A study at the 6th Convalescent Center reconfirmed Korean War findings that bed rest was not essential after the patient had recovered from the acute phase of this illness.

Recently, added attention has been paid to the serum hepatitis problem. Its true extent among American soldiers is unknown because it is masked by over-all hepatitis statistics, but those who ran the greatest risk were men receiving multiple transfusions after battle injury, and those injecting illicit drugs intravenously.

Diarrheal Diseases

The incidence of that fraction of diarrheal disease severe enough to require hospitalization or assignment to quarters showed a steady downward trend between 1965 and 1970. In 1965, the average theater-wide annual rate for this type of disease was 69 per 1,000 per year; in 1969, it was 35 per 1,000 per year. Also during this period, the difference between the annual high and low rates was significantly reduced, indicating an improvement in control during periods of peak disease incidence. In 1965, this difference was 55.4; in 1969, it was 18.7.

A comparison with World War II experience gives Vietnam diarrheal disease rates added significance. With respect to the China-Burma-India theater, it was reported that ". . . except for an occasional winter month, monthly rates for diarrheas and dysenteries were never under 100 per 1,000 per year until the fall of 1945." For both the China-Burma-India and Southwest Pacific theaters, average annual rates, when viewed over a period of time, did not reveal a downward trend as did those for Vietnam; furthermore, the Vietnam rate was a fraction of the rates for these areas. (*Table 4*) Accurate comparisons with the Korean experience cannot be made because of differences in the bases for statistics in the two conflicts.

Incidence of diarrheal disease peaked in May or June, corresponding with the monsoon season, and sometimes reached a secondary peak in October. (*Chart 10*) Affected most severely were unacclimatized troops and troops under combat conditions. For the latter, disease often stemmed from feces-laden soil being washed into inadequately protected water supplies in the field.

Any one of a host of viral, bacterial, or parasitic agents caused diarrhea in Vietnam; an exact etiology could not be identified in most instances. When specific agents were identified, excellent therapy was readily available. The average hospital stay for a patient with a diarrheal problem was 5½ days.

TABLE 4.—INCIDENCE RATE OF DIARRHEAL DISEASE AMONG U.S. ARMY PERSONNEL IN WORLD WAR II AND IN VIETNAM, BY YEAR

[Rate expressed as number of cases per annum per 1,000 average strength]

World War II			Vietnam	
Year	China-Burma-India Rate	Southwest Pacific Rate	Year	Rate
1942	123	59	1965	69
1943	146	70	1966	48
1944	181	55	1967	49
1945	93	74	1968	43
			1969	35

Sources: (1) World War II: Morbidity and Mortality in the United States Army, 1940–45. Preliminary Table Based on Periodic Summary Reports, Office of the Surgeon General, U.S. Army. (2) Vietnam: Health of the Army, May 1966, May 1967, May 1968, May 1969, May 1970, Office of the Surgeon General, U.S. Army.

CHART 10—ADMISSIONS TO HOSPITAL AND QUARTERS FOR DIARRHEAL DISEASE AMONG U.S. ARMY PERSONNEL IN VIETNAM, 1965–69

[Rate expressed as number of admissions per annum per 1,000 average strength]

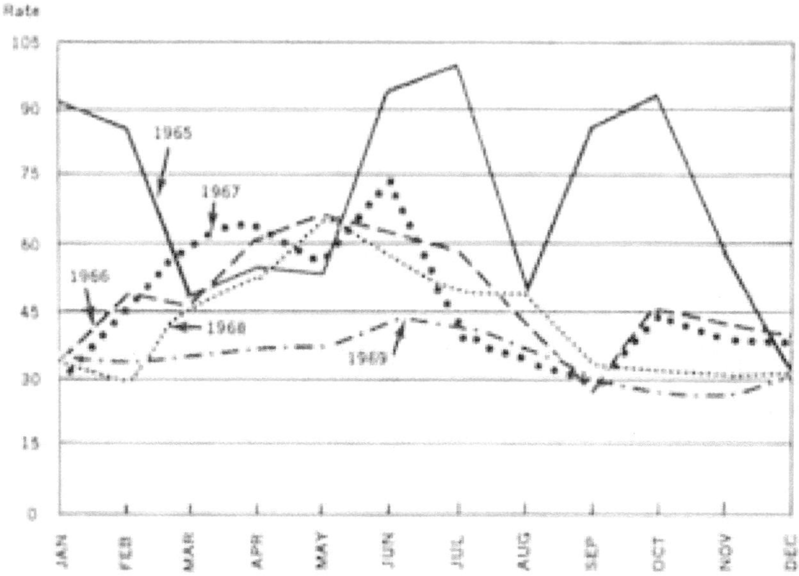

Source: Health of the Army, May 1966, May 1967, May 1968, May 1969, and May 1970. Office of the Surgeon General, United States Army.

It is notable that cholera, the most feared of diarrheal diseases, has not been a military problem in Vietnam, though it is endemic in the civilian population. Immunization against typhoid fever, however, has not been so effective; 25 Army cases have occurred in the theater, 13 of these in 1970.

Diseases of the Skin

Rates of incidence of skin disease severe enough to require hospitalization or admission to quarters in Vietnam varied around the 30 per 1,000 per year level until 1968, when the institution of a prophylactic program resulted in a dramatic drop to the 20 per 1,000 per year level. (*See Table 3.*) Figures for 1970, however, indicate a resurgence of this problem to heights comparable to those of 1965. This rise is, as yet, unexplained.

No adequate statistics exist for the comparison of dermatological problems in Vietnam with those of World War II and Korea. As previously noted, hospital statistics provide minimum figures only in this area of disease; dermatological problems have been severely debilitating in units operating in flooded areas of Vietnam.

The three major skin disease problems in Vietnam have been superficial fungal infection (dermatophytosis), bacterial infection, and immersion foot. Disease is probably due to the interaction of four factors: changes brought about in the resistance of the skin to infection because of prolonged exposure to contaminated water; damage to the skin by trauma and friction generated by wearing boots and socks; presence of the etiological organisms in the watery environment; and increased temperature of the tropical environment. Susceptibility to dermatological diseases increased with time in combat, peaking at the 10th month, although some individuals had inherent immunity. Black troops proved to be less susceptible than white troops.

The keynote in dealing with the militarily important dermatological diseases in Vietnam was prevention. Immersion foot was treated through the use of a drying-out period, and the others through the therapeutic use of griseofulvin-V, broadscope antibiotics, and a variety of topical treatments.

Melioidosis

Melioidosis, one of the more exotic medical problems encountered by U.S. troops in Vietnam, is an infectious disease caused by *Pseudomonas pseudomalli*, a common bacterium of Southeast Asia that has been cultured from soil, market fruits and vegetables, well water, and surface water. The source of the infection is not fully known, nor has man-to-man transference been observed.

In humans, melioidosis is manifest in one of three ways: by acute lung infection, by overwhelming systemic infection, or by localized abscess. The unfamiliarity of American physicians with this disease and their concomitant failure to diagnose and treat it properly in all but the most severe cases are shown in the low rate and high fatality incidence in 1966:

Year	*Cases*	*Deaths*
1965	6	0
1966	29	8
1967	50	3
1968	56	1
1969	46	1
1970	43	1

Although multiple antibiotics were initially used to treat melioidosis, it has become clear over time that tetracycline alone was the drug of choice. Since 1967, most patients have been treated and returned to duty in Vietnam. Patients evacuated from Vietnam or found to have the disease after departing were referred to Valley Forge General Hospital, Phoenixville, Pa., or Fitzsimons General Hospital, Denver, Colo., both designated by The Surgeon General as melioidosis treatment centers.

Neuropsychiatric Problems

Psychosis and neurosis. Until 1968, the neuropsychiatric disease rate in Vietnam remainded roughly stable and parallel with that for the rest of the Army. In that year, however, Army-wide rates began to increase, and rates in Vietnam increased more precipitously than in any other location where substantial numbers of American troops were serving. (*Table 5, Chart 11*) Rising rates showed increases in all areas of psychiatric illness: psychosis, psychoneurosis, character and behavior disorders, for example.

CHART 11—ADMISSIONS TO HOSPITAL AND QUARTERS FOR NEUROPSYCHIATRIC CONDITIONS (PSYCHOTIC, PSYCHONEUROTIC, AND CHARACTER AND BEHAVIOR DISORDERS) AMONG U.S. ARMY PERSONNEL IN VIETNAM, 1965–69

[Rate expressed as number of admissions per annum per 1,000 average strength]

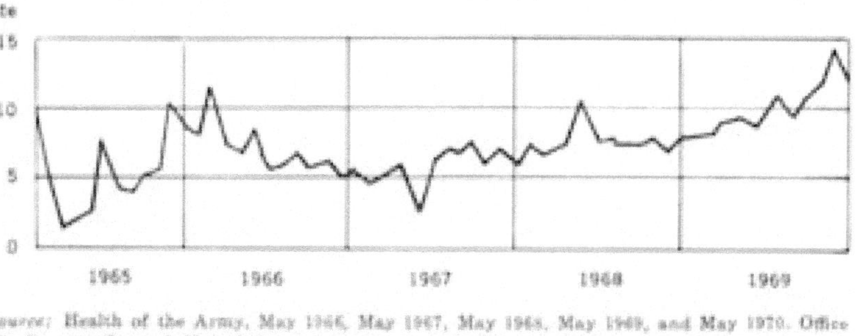

Source: Health of the Army, May 1966, May 1967, May 1968, May 1969, and May 1970. Office of the Surgeon General, United States Army.

The extent of the problem is evident from several statistical indices. Rates for admission to hospital and quarters for neuropsychiatric cases in Vietnam more than doubled between 1965 (11.7 per 1,000 per year) and 1970 (25.1 per 1,000 per year). (*See Table 3.*) In terms of estimated man-days lost, neuropsychiatric conditions were the second leading disease problem in the theater in 1970; the 175,510 figure for that year is more than twice as high as the estimate for 1967 (70,000), reflecting a steady increase over the 1967–70 period. (*See Table 2.*)

Statistics in this area are not comparable with those for World War II and Korea because of differences in diagnostic standards and categories, but it is notable that, unlike the case for World War II, in Viet-

TABLE 5.—INCIDENCE RATE OF PSYCHIATRIC CONDITIONS, ARMY-WIDE, 1965–70

[Rate expressed as number of cases per annum per 1,000 average strength]

Year	Total psychiatric conditions				Psychosis				Psychoneurosis			
	Army-wide	CONUS	USAREUR	RVN	Army-wide	CONUS	USAREUR	RVN	Army-wide	CONUS	USAREUR	RVN
1965	9. 1	9. 1	7. 7	10. 8	1. 4	1. 6	0. 7	1. 6	1. 6	1. 5	1. 0	2. 3
1966	10. 3	10. 8	7. 3	11. 6	1. 7	2. 1	0. 8	1. 4	1. 9	2. 0	1. 0	2. 5
1967	9. 7	9. 5	8. 2	9. 8	1. 6	1. 8	0. 9	1. 7	1. 7	1. 9	1. 0	1. 3
1968	10. 3	9. 9	7. 9	12. 7	1. 8	1. 9	0. 9	1. 8	1. 9	1. 9	1. 2	2. 2
1969	11. 3	10. 4	7. 8	15. 1	2. 6	2. 4	1. 6	3. 4	1. 7	1. 6	1. 5	1. 9
1970 [1]	15. 4	12. 5	9. 7	24. 0	3. 3	3. 2	2. 4	3. 8	2. 3	1. 9	1. 8	3. 3

Year	Character and behavior disorders				Other psychiatric conditions			
	Army-wide	CONUS	USAREUR	RVN	Army-wide	CONUS	USAREUR	RVN
1965	2. 3	2. 0	2. 2	3. 1	3. 8	4. 0	3. 8	3. 8
1966	2. 5	2. 4	2. 2	2. 8	4. 2	4. 3	3. 3	4. 9
1967	2. 4	2. 1	2. 2	2. 9	4. 0	3. 7	4. 1	3. 9
1968	2. 3	1. 8	1. 8	3. 7	4. 3	4. 3	4. 0	5. 0
1969	2. 4	1. 8	1. 6	4. 2	4. 6	4. 6	3. 1	5. 6
1970 [1]	3. 7	1. 7	1. 9	8. 4	6. 1	5. 7	3. 6	8. 5

[1] January–September only.

Source: Morbidity Report, RCS MED–78.

nam the incidence of neuropsychiatric admissions did not co-vary with the incidence of combat injury. Rather, neuropsychiatric rates rose despite the diminishing combat role in that country in 1969 and 1970.

Several hypotheses have been offered to explain these rising rates in the Army in general and in Vietnam in particular. It has been suggested, for example, that increased drug abuse has been reflected in increased rates of psychosis, rates which include toxic (drug-induced) psychosis. For Vietnam, it has also been suggested that identity with another peer group, such as one based upon race, political affiliation, or drug use, at the unit level has threatened the integrity of the squad as the sole reference point for the soldier in combat. This tendency in turn resulted in rising neuropsychiatric rates among individuals who, presented with alternatives, lack the certainty in the stress of combat that confidence in the squad gave the World War II infantryman. These and other hypotheses are currently under study.

In providing psychiatric support for combat troops, the practice in Vietnam was to offer aid as close to the unit as possible, relying upon the social worker and enlisted clinical specialist, and upon three basic tools: rest, sedation, and supportive psychotherapy. Guidelines indicated that hospitalization was to be avoided except when the patient was dangerous to himself or others or mentally ill. Hospitalization for simple drunkenness, for sociopathological individuals, or for administrative convenience was forbidden by regulation. This adds significance to the rising statistics cited previously.

Drug abuse. One of the unique problems that faced the Medical Department in Vietnam was the drug milieu into which the American soldier was immersed, both on and off duty, upon arrival in the theater. The growth of illicit drug use within the Army kept pace with that in the larger society, but the ready availability of marijuana, barbiturates, amphetamines, heroin, opium, and other substances in Vietnam, at a lower price for a less adulterated product than that available in the United States, exacerbated the problem.

Comprehensive statistics are not available, but preliminary work based upon sample surveys of soldiers entering and leaving the combat zone indicates that illegal drug use is widespread, especially among younger, lower ranking enlisted men, and that many individuals started using drugs while in Vietnam. One study, done in 1969 at the Cam Ranh Bay replacement depot by Captain Morris Stanton, MC, reported that, of a population of 994 outgoing enlisted men, 53.2 percent had tried marijuana sometime in their lives, 21.5 percent for the first time in Vietnam. The same study reported that the use of opium among the soldiers sampled nearly tripled during their stay in Vietnam, rising from 6.3 percent to 17.4 percent.

Growing command awareness of the nature and extent of the drug problem in Vietnam led to a search for a flexible, nonpunitive response that would encourage drug users to seek professional help in solving their problems, thus aiding them and, at the same time, serve the Army's interest in conserving the fighting strength. This search resulted in a two-fold program in Vietnam. At the first level the program was educational, bringing information about the problem to key commissioned and non-commissioned officers so that they could deal intelligently with it, and provide believable advice about drug abuse to the troops in Vietnam. The latter task was the more difficult because conflicting information available in all sectors of American society about the dangers of marijuana and the linking of its use with other drug problems led to a state of incredulity among American troops. This credibility gap was partially overcome through the use of ex-addicts in information programs, through the realistic redirection of the efforts of the Armed Forces Radio, and through an attempt to dispense factual data personally through medical channels.

But informational activities were directed at men who had not yet become deeply involved with drugs. For others less fortunate, the experimental institution of an amnesty program in the 4th Infantry Division in 1968 attracted wide attention as a promising attempt to deal with the problem. The program provided that a soldier who voluntarily presented himself as a drug user to his commanding officer, chaplain, or unit surgeon, would not be punished merely for admitting to the use of drugs, if this use had not previously come to the attention of the command. The drug user who voluntarily sought assistance was aided through limited hospitalization to determine the nature and extent of his addiction; through extensive psychiatric and other counseling, including group therapy when possible; and through assignment of a "buddy" to give him positive reinforcement in his effort to give up drugs. During the period of counseling and rehabilitation, the patient continued, as much as possible, to perform full military duties. The 4th Infantry Division's program was adopted throughout the Army in December 1970.

CHAPTER III

Care of the Wounded*

Excellence of Medical Care

Factors in Low Morbidity and Mortality

The excellence of care of the wounded in Vietnam was the result of a combination of factors: rapid evacuation of the casualty, ready availability of whole blood, well-established forward hospitals, advanced surgical techniques, and improved medical management.

From the standpoint of methods used to wound—mines, high-velocity missiles, and boobytraps—as well as the locale in which many were injured—in paddy fields or along waterways where human and animal excreta were common—Vietnam was quite a "dirty" war. Yet helicopters were able to evacuate most casualties to medical facilities before a serious wound could become worse. There were practically no conditions under which the injured was denied timely evacuation; weather, terrain, time of day, enemy contact, all were surmounted by the capabilities of the air ambulances and the skill of their crews.

The use of whole blood, occasionally even before the arrival of an air ambulance, contributed to the low mortality rate in Vietnam by better preparing the wounded for evacuation. Blood packaged in styrofoam containers which permitted storage for 48 to 72 hours in the field could be placed in the forward area in anticipation of casualties. This was a marked increase in the utilization of whole blood, since virtually none was used at the division level in World War II. Stocks of blood, drawn from PACOM (Pacific Command) in the early years and later

*This chapter, involved with statistical analysis of World War II, Korea, and Vietnam as indices of the quality of care of the wounded, is subject to all the handicaps of comparison. Reporting procedures have changed over the last 25 years, and the most recent reports included more individuals through the increased scope and efficiency of the data collecting system; moreover, some information gathered for Vietnam had no true counterpart in the previous conflicts. Yet another problem is semantics: "hospitals" is different from "all medical treatment facilities," which presents the danger of "comparing" what is actually two different populations. Concern with these problems is highly justified, and any reader must view comparisons merely as illustration of trends, not as absolute fact. While the figures will change as more complete information becomes available, the basic fact which they illuminate will not—the care of the wounded in Vietnam has been superior to that given in combat anywhere at anytime.

largely from CONUS (continental United States), were always sufficient.

The relative stability of forward hospitals in Vietnam made possible the use of sophisticated equipment. Air conditioning to counter the extreme heat, dust, and humidity allowed better control of the environment of the wounded before, during, and after surgery, and was necessary for the proper functioning of the highly sensitive equipment. Commenting on hospital apparatus, the USARV neurosurgical consultant, Lieutenant Colonel Robert C. Leaver, MC, stated, "The traditional equipment seen in neurosurgical centers throughout the United States is available, i.e., respirators, Stryker frames, and hypothermia units. Other than the physical deficiencies of a hospital in a combat area, there is little that would distinguish our neurosurgical wards from those in hospitals in America."

Surgical technique as practiced in Vietnam was certainly as advanced as the state of the art in general, and perhaps more so in the realm of trauma. Contrary to traditional procedure, surgeons in Vietnam rediscovered that wounds (except cranial and facial, and some hand injuries) responded better to a delayed closure which permitted necessary drainage. Management of severe liver injury was a real therapeutic challenge since massive transfusion, control of relatively inaccessible bleeding, and removal of large portions of liver substance were often required. Surgeons performed complex operations daily and routinely in all hospitals, not just selected ones in the rear. Vascular surgery, sporadic in Korea, was commonplace in Vietnam, and surgeons became so adept that not only thoracic but also general and orthopedic surgeons routinely performed repairs.

The high level of skill was maintained despite the turnover of medical officers. Since surgeons arriving in Vietnam were not adequately prepared by their background in civil trauma to treat combat casualties, they were attached to experienced teams for orientation and learned technique in the operating room.

Improved medical management of the casualty contributed to the quality care. Surgery itself had become a part of the continuing process of resuscitation and a weapon in the struggle against shock. The team approach, in which surgeons of a variety of specialties operated together, also proved highly effective; a "team" for head injuries, for example, included a neurosurgeon, ophthalmologist, oral surgeon, otolaryngologist, and plastic surgeon. If the casualty had multiple injuries, more than one surgical team operated simultaneously.

Survival Statistics

Between January 1965 and December 1970, 133,447 wounded were admitted to medical treatment facilities in Vietnam; 97,659 of these were admitted to hospitals. The hospital mortality rate for this period was 2.6

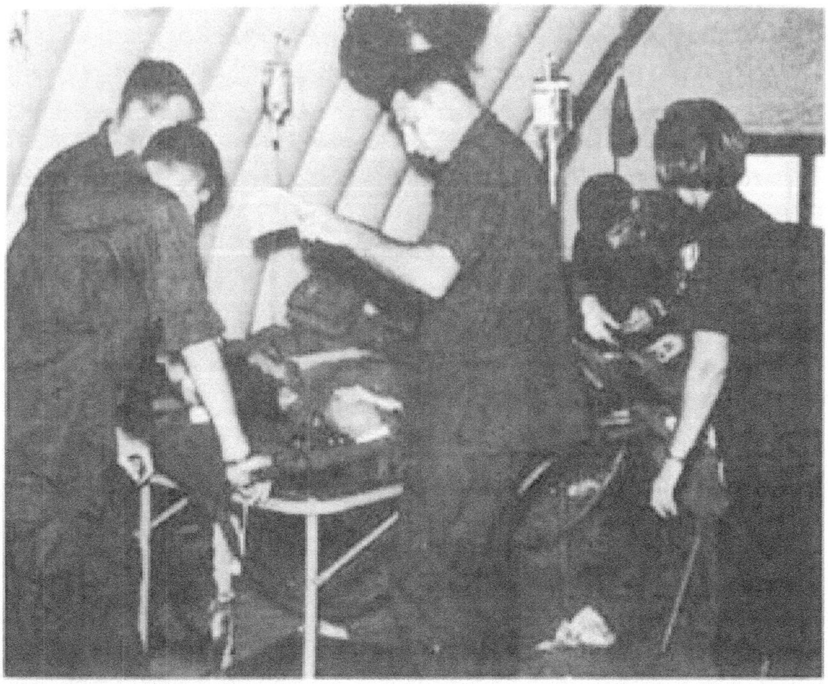

A WOUNDED AMERICAN SOLDIER RECEIVES IMMEDIATE TREATMENT *upon arrival at a MUST field hospital in Vietnam.*

percent, compared to 4.5 percent in World War II and 2.5 percent in Korea. The very slight increase in hospital mortality in Vietnam over that in Korea was a result of rapid helicopter evacuation which brought into the hospital mortally wounded patients who, with earlier, slower means of evacuation, would have died en route and would have been recorded as KIA (killed in action). Assuming that most of those patients who died within the first 24 hours in hospitals belong in this class, the rate would be much closer to 1 percent. Actually, it is further testimony to the high quality of medical care provided in Vietnam where even though mortally wounded casualties arrived at Army hospitals, the mortality rate was only marginally greater than in Korea.

Perhaps a better index of the effectiveness of medical treatment was the ratio of deaths to deaths plus surviving wounded (or "deaths as a percent of hits"). For World War II, it was 29.3 percent; Korea, 26.3 percent; and Vietnam, 19.0 percent. The ratio of KIA to WIA (wounded in action) was as follows: World War II, 1:3.1; Korea, 1:4.1; Vietnam, 1:5.6.

Patient Care Indices

Since the task of the combat physician is to salvage as much limb or function as possible, and the goal of the Medical Department is the salvage of lives, it is proper that the accomplishments of the Medical Department mission in Vietnam be measured in terms of lives recovered rather than numbers lost.

The bed occupancy rate in Vietnam ran approximately 60 percent, and that in offshore facilities about 50 percent, which allowed ample flexibility to respond to fluctuating casualty rates and remain capable of providing optimum medical care.

The average length of stay per case for patients in Vietnam was considerably below that of both earlier conflicts:

	Days
World War II . . .	80
Korean War	75
Vietnam*	63

*Through July 1967.

This reduction of approximately 20 percent reflected the advances in wound management and patient care.

Of the 194,716 wounded in Vietnam (January 1965–December 1970), 61,269 (31 percent) were treated and returned to duty immediately. Of those admitted to treatment facilities, the distribution was as follows:

42.1 percent returned to duty in RVN
7.6 percent returned to duty in PACOM
33.4 percent returned to duty in CONUS
2.7 percent still hospitalized, 31 December 1970
14.2 percent other dispositions (died; transferred to Veterans' Administration hospital; discharged; and so forth)

Two to three percent of the hospitalized wounded in Vietnam had significant vascular injuries, and the amputation rate for those with major arterial injury was about 13 percent. This rate was approximately the same as that for Korea, and markedly less than the 49 percent rate for World War II. The approach was for maximum conservation of stump length which, in conjunction with developments in prosthetic manufacture, decreased morbidity and length of hospitalization among orthopedic patients.

Nature of Wounds

The lethality of modern weapons directly affected the work of the medical personnel who attempted to undo the damage. While one must be wary of dubbing things "new," certainly the problems which medical personnel in Vietnam encountered were more complicated than before.

Mechanics of Wounding

High-velocity, lightweight rounds from M16/AK47-type weapons have greater kinetic energy and leave larger temporary and permanent cavities and more severe tissue damage than do low-velocity projectiles, and their easy deflection by foliage resulted in tumbling and spinning and the generation of even larger entrance wounds. Moreover, blood vessels not in the direct path of the missile were affected. The bullet usually disintegrated and was rarely found whole even when an exit wound was absent. These rapid fire weapons increased the chances of multiple wounding, which complicated resuscitation and treatment.

The claymore mine received its first field trials by both sides in Vietnam. The intensity of peppering and velocity of the fragments often resulted in deep penetration in a number of sites. The extensive use of mines and boobytraps in Vietnam created a serious medical problem: the proximity of the blast caused severe local destruction, and tremendous amounts of dirt, debris, and secondary missiles were hurled into the wound. Massive contamination challenged the surgeon to choose between radical excision of potentially salvageable tissue and a more conservative approach which might leave a source of infection.

Causative Agents

The data on the physical agents which caused wounds and deaths reflect the nature of the combat. Much higher proportions of the casualties were caused by small arms fire, and by boobytraps and mines, than in Korea or World War II, and much lower percentages were caused by artillery and other explosive projectile fragments. This relationship generally was more pronounced among the fatalities than among the wounded. (*Table 6*)

Statistics compiled at different times in the Vietnam conflict mirrored the shift in combat from the defensive to the offensive. In 1965, U.S. forces were most concerned with establishing and defending their bases, and only in 1966 did they launch operations to check the enemy offensive. By 1968, troops were usually engaging the enemy in his defensive positions. Wounding from small arms fire decreased from 42.7 percent in June 1966 to 16 percent in June 1970, while the percentage from fragments (including mines and boobytraps) rose from 49.6 percent in 1966 to 80 percent in 1970.

TABLE 6.—PERCENT OF DEATHS AND WOUNDS ACCORDING TO AGENT, U.S. ARMY, IN THREE WARS: WORLD WAR II, KOREA, AND VIETNAM

Agent	Deaths			Wounds		
	World War II	Korea	Vietnam [1]	World War II	Korea	Vietnam [1]
Small arms	32	33	51	20	27	16
Fragments	53	59	36	62	61	65
Booby traps, mines	3	4	11	4	4	15
Punji stakes						2
Other	12	4	2	14	8	2

[1] January 1965–June 1970.

Source: Statistical Data on Army Troops Wounded in Vietnam, January 1965–June 1970, Medical Statistics Agency, Office of the Surgeon General, U.S. Army.

Anatomical Location of Wounds

The rapid fire weapons of the enemy resulted in a significant increase over World War II and Korea in the percentages of multiple wounds among the distribution of wounds by site. (*Table 7*)

Small arms fire caused approximately two-thirds of the wounds of the head and neck, and three-fourths of the trunk wounds; fragments accounted for the remainder. Fragments and small arms contributed fairly equally to wounds of the extremities.

The distribution of fatal wounds by location differed from that for total wounds since some areas were much more likely to involve mortal

TABLE 7.—LOCATION OF WOUNDS IN HOSPITALIZED CASUALTIES, BY PERCENT, U.S. ARMY, IN THREE WARS: WORLD WAR II, KOREA, AND VIETNAM

Anatomical location	World War II	Korea	Vietnam [1]
Head and neck	17	17	14
Thorax	7	7	7
Abdomen	8	7	5
Upper extremities	25	30	18
Lower extremities	40	37	36
Other sites	3	2	[2]20

[1] For a 24-month period.

[2] Including multiple wounds.

Source: Statistical Data on Army Troops Wounded in Vietnam, January 1965–June 1970, Medical Statistics Agency, Office of the Surgeon General, U.S. Army.

injuries than others. Thus the 14 percent of the wounds located in the head and neck region accounted for 39 percent of the fatalities. This was followed by 19.3 percent fatal wounds in the thorax; 17.9 percent, abdomen; 16.1 percent, multiple sites; 6.8 percent, lower extremities; and 0.9 percent, upper extremities. Twenty to thirty percent of the penetrating head wounds brought in from the field in Vietnam were classed as "expectant" cases, and little could have been done for them; however, the mortality rate for the others was rather low because of early evacuation, extensive use of blood, and the presence of fully trained neurosurgeons in the combat zone. Most of the abdominal fatalities were from extensive liver destruction or multiple organ involvement.

Certainly the data on relative lethality of wounds and the distribution by causative agent showed the advantage of wearing properly designed body armor. Had helmets been worn, they would have proved very effective against fragments, although little could be done in the event of a direct hit by a small arms round. To quote Lieutenant Colonel (later Colonel) William M. Hammon, MC: "If our combat troops . . . were to wear the helmet, we believe that about ⅓ fewer significant combat casualties would need to be admitted to a neurosurgical center here in Vietnam." Flak vests did prove effective against three-fourths of the fragments which struck the thorax, thereby increasing the percentage of gunshot wounds to other areas of the body to 75 percent of chest wounds.

Troops in static positions, or in air or ground vehicles, usually wore both helmets and flak vests, but soldiers on the move found the body armor too heavy and too hot. Some commanders (and some individuals regardless of the command decision) decided to forego the protection rather than accept the reduction in mission capability and the increase in heat casualties.

Specific Advances

The continuous thrust of the U.S. Army Medical Department in combat surgery is on the development of better procedures and ancillary techniques for the care of the wounded. In Vietnam, concern centered on the areas of anesthesia, blood and plasma expanders, treatment of burns, wound healing, shock, and surgical routine.

Anesthesia

Most surgery in Vietnam hospitals was done under a general anesthetic, usually thiopental induction and maintenance with halothane, nitrous oxide, and oxygen. Most anesthesiologists favored halothane, with its rapid action, ease of administration, nonflammability and applicability to all cases; also, it did not produce nausea and did not mask critical drops in blood volume.

Local anesthetics were used only for very minor wounds and a few delayed primary closures. Employment of spinal anesthesia was very limited. The emphasis continued on development of safe, simplified methods of portable inhalation anesthesia.

New concepts for assisting the breathing of the critically injured were also developed to meet Vietnam requirements. Prolonged mechanical support was necessary in some cases to minimize oxygen deficiency, and while respirators were ordinarily used, the possibility existed that harmful bacteria might be introduced since proper sterilization was not always feasible under combat conditions. New respiratory assistance devices, eliminating or reducing that potentiality, were tested.

Blood and Plasma Expanders

Frequently transfusions of whole blood were initiated long before the casualty reached a facility with the capacity for cross-matching blood, and in these cases, type O low titer blood was used. As a rule, any patient who had received four or more units of type O low titer was continued on this type, while those with less than four were matched at the hospital.

Massive transfusions (one surviving patient had received 92 units), although lifesaving, presented problems of their own. A tendency toward bleeding appeared after multiple transfusions, but it was found that fresh frozen plasma or, if possible, freshly drawn blood could control the condition. Also, the patient whose body temperature dropped as a result of extensive transfusion became a serious problem. Two evacuation hospitals utilized microwave ovens to warm the whole unit of blood in seconds to counter this condition.

Burns

The most unfortunate aspect of the burn injuries incurred in Vietnam was that more than half were accidental and therefore preventable. Burns associated with enemy fire, while fewer in number, accounted for almost 70 percent of the fatalities because of their severity and associated wounds. A factor in the high mortality was that most combat burns occurred in an enclosed space, such as an armored personnel carrier or a bunker, and were, therefore, complicated by inhalation injuries.

Burn cases were stabilized in-country and then evacuated to the 106th General Hospital in Japan, where a special burn unit had been established. Of the burns treated by the 106th, 27 percent returned to duty, 66 percent were evacuated to the burn unit at Brooke Army Medical Center, Fort Sam Houston, Tex., and 7 percent died.

Sulfamylon ointment was employed to prevent infection. If evacuation to Japan was delayed more than 48 hours, treatment was initiated in Vietnam. Since the standard treatment of phosphorus burns with copper sulfate solution was found to be toxic in itself, their management became even more difficult and debridement of the wound grew more important.

Wound Healing

The Surgical Research Team, WRAIR (Walter Reed Army Institute of Research), tested in Vietnam several experimental items developed to aid wound healing. An antibiotic preparation, packaged as an aerosol, was distributed to aidmen in various tactical units. Immediate use on an open wound acted to retard bacteria growth, and resulted in decreased morbidity. Tissue adhesives which had low toxicity, degraded relatively rapidly, and spread well proved valuable in surgery on the lung, kidneys, and liver. The Surgical Research Team utilized them with excellent results as early as 1968.

Shock

Shock was a killer which was checked somewhat by the rapid evacuation system and the whole blood available to the wounded in Vietnam. Yet even so, mortality rates were increased by a postoperative pulmonary complication known as shock lung or wet lung where the lung or thorax had been traumatized. By the time the condition could be detected by X-ray, it was usually too advanced to respond to treatment. However, after extensive investigation, Colonel James P. Geiger, MC, surgical consultant from June 1969 to June 1970, identified the mechanics of the problem and demonstrated that the complication could be forestalled by the use of diuretics in those likely to be so afflicted. This treatment significantly reduced the morbidity and mortality in the syndrome.

Surgical Routine

An outstanding feature of medical service in Vietnam was the quality and extent of care given in the battle area. Any type of medical or surgical specialist was available in the combat zone. For example, by the spring of 1968, there were 10 neurosurgeons at five Army hospitals, supervised by a board-certified neurosurgeon.

Sophisticated operations were handled as a matter of routine. Laparotomies were done "on suspicion" (which proved positive in about 25 percent of the cases) in a zone where heretofore there was a degree of reluctance to operate even when abdominal penetration was certain. Primary repairs were performed on veins which had simply been ligated in earlier conflicts, and fasciotomy, cutting the tissue sheathing the muscles and reducing pressure on the muscles, was not uncommon. In a few instances, limb salvage was possible by constructing an extra anatomic bypass, tunneling a graft through a new route around the area, until the wound healed and a permanent vascular graft could be inserted. The expert surgeon, supported by a skilled medical team and well-equipped facilities, provided a quality of care superior to that in any previous conflict.

CHAPTER IV

Hospitalization and Evacuation

The peculiar nature of counterinsurgency operations in Vietnam required modification of the usual concepts of hospital usage in a combat area. There was no "front" in the tradition of World War II. The Army checkered the countryside with base camps. Although any one of these might become a battlefield, the base camp was relatively secure unless it was under attack. Semipermanent, air-conditioned, fully equipped hospitals were constructed at a number of these camps. In contrast to World War II and the Korean War, the hospital did not follow the advancing army in direct support of tactical operations. All Army hospitals in Vietnam, including the MUST (Medical Unit, Self-contained, Transportable) units, were fixed installations with area support missions. Since there was no secure road network in the combat area of Vietnam, surface evacuation of the wounded was almost impossible. Use of the five separate companies and five detachments of ground ambulances sent to Vietnam was limited largely to such functions at base camps as transportation between the landing strip and the hospital or the routine transfer of patients between neighboring hospitals when roads were secure. Air evacuation of the injured became routine.

Getting the casualty and the physician together as soon as possible is the keystone of the practice of combat medicine. The helicopter achieved this goal as never before. Of equal importance was that the Medical Department was getting the two together in a hospital environment equipped to meet almost any situation. The degree of sophistication of medical equipment and facilities everywhere in Vietnam permitted Army physicians to make full use of their training and capability. As a result, the care that was available in Army hospitals in Vietnam was far better than any that had ever been generally available for combat support. The technical development of the helicopter ambulance, a primitive version of which had been used to a limited extent in the Korean War, the growth of a solid body of doctrine on air evacuation procedures, and the skill, ingenuity, and courage of the aircraft crewmen and medical aidmen who put theory into practice in a hostile and dangerous environment made possible the hospitalization and evacuation system that evolved in Vietnam. The system worked effectively because it was compatible with the characteristics of warfare in that country.

Hospitalization

Until April 1965, the 8th Field Hospital at Nha Trang with a 100-bed capacity was the only U.S. Army hospital in Vietnam. Housed in fixed semipermanent quarters, the 8th Field was fitted with a combination of field and "stateside" equipment and operated in a manner similar to a station hospital. Attached to it were four medical detachments which provided specialty care but were totally dependent on the hospital for administrative and logistical support.

In October 1963, the Navy opened a dispensary in Saigon which removed that city, as well as III and IV CTZ's to the south, from the hospitalization responsibility of the 8th Field Hospital. It remained responsible only for the large area encompassed by II CTZ.

Because of the limited number of Army hospital beds in Vietnam to support the buildup of U.S. combat forces in 1965, a variable 15- to 30-day evacuation policy was established by the Surgeon, USMACV. By mid-1966, the number of beds had increased sufficiently to permit a change to a 30-day policy. Patients who could be treated and returned to duty within 30 days were retained in Vietnam; patients requiring hospitalization for a longer period were evacuated out-of-country as soon as their medical condition permitted.

In the development of the medical troop list, the length of the evacuation policy did not weigh as heavily as the patient treatment capability required in-country. Among the factors which affected the normal book planning of allocations were the lack of data on the number and types of foreseeable casualties in counterinsurgency operations, the insecure ground lines of communication, and the wide separation of secure base areas. No single factor had as great an influence in determining the number of hospital beds required as the policy approved by USMACV to keep 40 percent of the operational beds available to support unexpected surges in the casualty flow resulting from hostile actions. The occupancy rate exceeded 60 percent on two occasions: during May 1967 when it briefly approached 67 percent, and for a 24-hour period during the Tet Offensive in February 1968, when it again increased to more than 65 percent.

Between April 1965 when the 3d Field Hospital arrived in Saigon and December of that year, two surgical hospitals, two evacuation hospitals, and several numbered field hospital units, which were initially colocated with the 8th Field Hospital in Nha Trang and the 3d Field Hospital in Saigon, were deployed to Vietnam. By the end of 1965, the total number of hospital beds in-country had increased to 1,627.

Throughout 1965, separate clearing companies were at times used interchangeably with hospitals. Augmented by specialty teams, platoons of these companies often preceded or supplanted hospitals, providing limited care within an area until more adequately staffed and equipped units arrived. Field-army-level clearing units were also used to augment hospitals and provide additional bed space. Dispensaries sometimes supplemented the resources of major hospitals and at other times provided outpatient service in remote areas.

The deployment of additional hospitals to Vietnam continued throughout 1966 and 1967. During 1966 and 1967, four surgical hospitals, six evacuation hospitals, and another hospital unit of a field hospital arrived in-country. The 6th Convalescent Center was established at Cam Ranh Bay.

The buildup of medical units was completed in 1968 with the arrival of one surgical hospital, three evacuation hospitals, and additional field hospital units, as well as 11 Reserve and National Guard medical units. The 312th Evacuation Hospital, the largest Reserve medical unit sent to Vietnam, arrived in September 1968, and occupied a facility the 2d Surgical Hospital had operated at Chu Lai. By December 1968, there were 5,283 Army hospital beds in Vietnam at facilities located throughout the four corps tactical zones. (*Map 2*)

With the exception of the 2d Surgical Hospital which moved from An Khe to Chu Lai on 8 May 1967 to support Task Force OREGON, the movement of hospitals was minimal before 1968. The problems encountered by the 22d Surgical Hospital in its move from Da Nang to Phu Bai were illustrative of the difficulties of moving medical facilities in the Vietnamese environment. The hospital was moved by LST (landing ship, tank) from Saigon to Da Nang. Enemy activity closed the road between Da Nang and Phu Bai, stranding the unit for several days while it awaited air transportation. The number of sorties required to complete the movement resulted in an even further delay.

The policy which called for minimal movement of hospitals was modified somewhat in 1968 and, to a greater extent, in 1969. The 22d Surgical Hospital and other medical units were sent to Phu Bai. The 18th Surgical Hospital was moved to Quang Tri, to Camp Evans, and back to Quang Tri. The 17th Field Hospital departed Saigon to operate in An Khe. The 27th Surgical Hospital was sent to Chu Lai after it came in-country, while the 95th Evacuation Hospital functioned in two different parts of Da Nang. The 29th Evacuation Hospital was established at Binh Thuy to support operations in the Delta, but was later deactivated and its facilities taken over by the 3d Surgical Hospital after it had moved from Dong Tam. The 91st Evacuation Hospital went to Chu Lai after the unit had built a facility near Tuy Hoa. The 85th Evacuation Hospital departed Qui Nhon for Phu Bai.

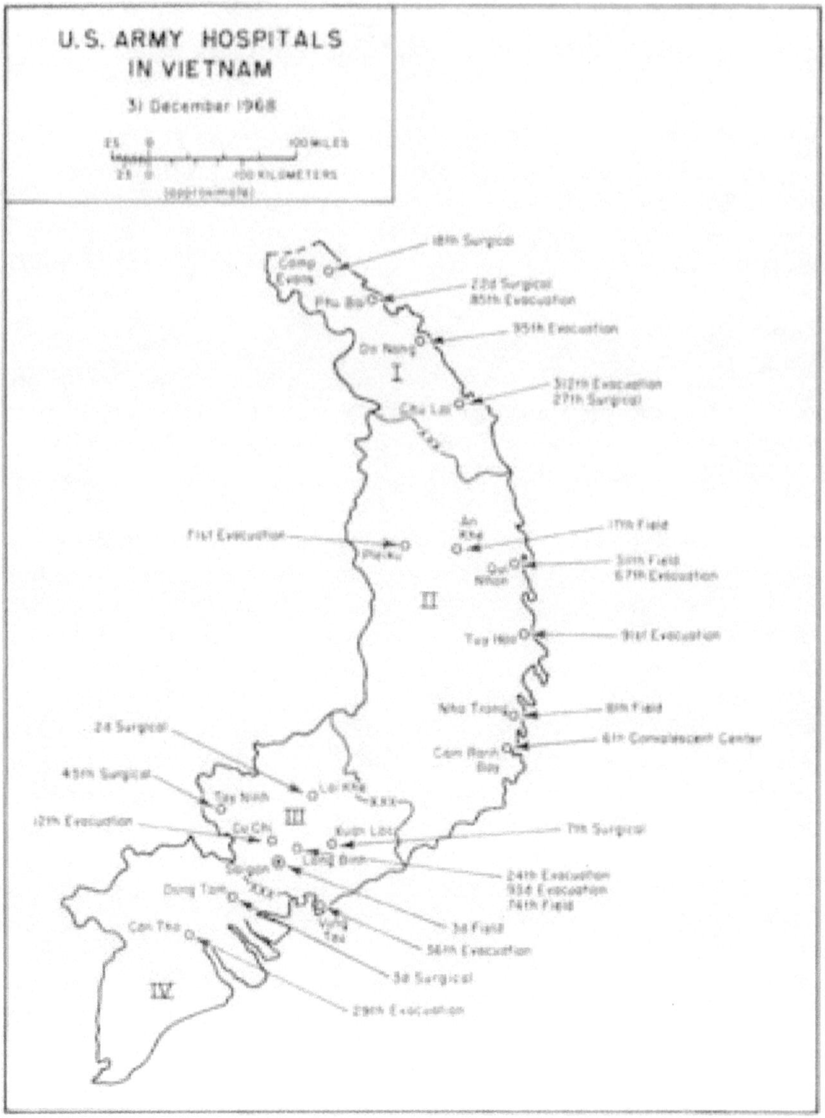

Map 2

Among other moves, the 2d Surgical Hospital remained temporarily at Chu Lai, then selected personnel deployed to Phu Bai to operate a 100-bed U.S. Army hospital (provisional) in facilities previously operated by the Marines. The provisional hospital was opened to retain the real estate and provide continued medical coverage in Phu Bai until a larger hospital could be constructed. When the 85th Evacuation Hospital took over in Phu Bai, the 2d Surgical Hospital moved to Lai Khe.

To a certain extent these moves were made to support increased Army combat activity in I CTZ and elsewhere, but they were not in support of tactical operations in the tradition of World War II and the Korean War. Except for the interim use of MUST equipment or existent buildings, the moves were made into semipermanent construction and were far more deliberate and complicated than the movement of tent-housed hospitals in previous conflicts. To a far greater extent shifts in 1968 and 1969 were the result of the deactivation of units and the consolidation of areas of support.

Construction

The construction of a modern hospital is a lengthy and complicated process. Line officers, medical staff planners, and hospital commanders soon found that many time-consuming, frustrating problems had to be resolved before construction could start.

Real estate was generally acquired in large sections for military use and then parceled out to the units needing it. Negotiations for a hospital site were often protracted. For example, the need for an evacuation hospital in the Pleiku area was recognized long before the area was secure enough to permit construction. Meanwhile, the original allocation of land for this use had been lost, and new negotiations were opened with the commander of the Vietnamese II Corps and the U.S. Air Force. It was some time before an agreement for suitable land was again reached and the contractor could begin work on the 71st Evacuation Hospital.

Hospitals were built in a wide variety of configurations, and construction was accomplished in almost as many ways as there were hospitals. Some structures, for example, the 91st Evacuation Hospital at Tuy Hoa, were built almost entirely by medical personnel with some technical advice from the Corps of Engineers. Some were started by contractors and finished by the Corps of Engineers. Medical personnel did some phase of the construction work in almost all the hospitals, but some work by contractors or engineers was needed in almost all cases to put in wiring, electrical fixtures, and heavy equipment.

In October 1965, the USARV surgeon and engineer established a policy for space utilization and prepared guidelines to govern hospital construction. This policy was disseminated in a USARV regulation which stated that patient wards, operating suites, and X-ray facilities were to be located in air-conditioned semipermanent structures. The use of these structures for medical purposes was to take precedence over that for troop billets, recreational areas, and administrative sections.

The improvement of existing medical facilities as well as the construction of new units continued to receive much attention during 1966 and 1967. Strict controls were placed on construction, and the position

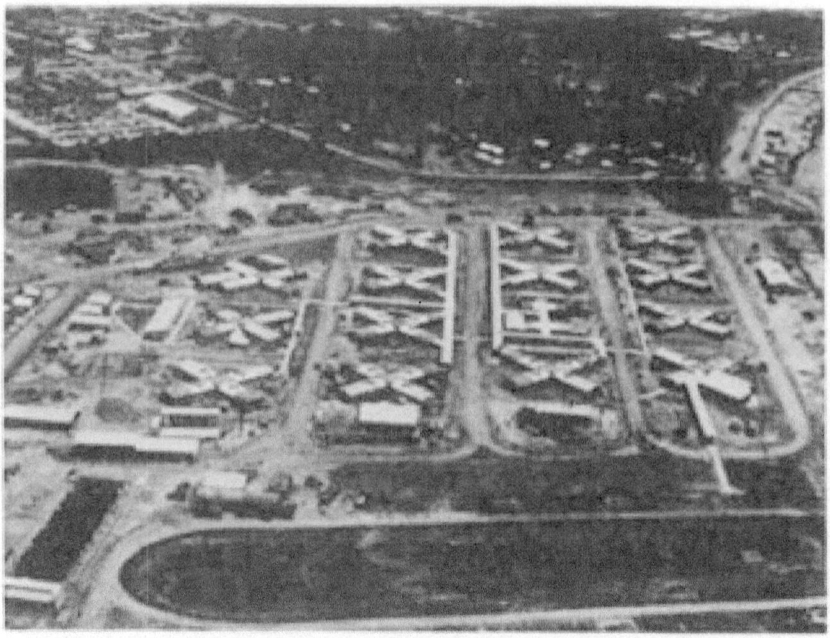

HOSPITALS IN VIETNAM, 1967

of base development co-ordinator was established at USARV headquarters. The base development co-ordinator was to evaluate the condition of hospitals and other medical treatment facilities, determine construction requirements, establish priorities, and limit or stop construction projects if duplication of effort was disclosed. Hospital construction was assigned a priority second only to the requirements of tactical units and communication centers.

The construction of dispensaries and dental clinics was given a lower priority. Adequate control had been established over the construction of army-level (separate) dispensaries, general dispensaries, and dental clinics, but control over the construction of unit dispensaries was initially inadequate. Some units constructed elaborate facilities, often located adjacent to another dispensary or hospital. Controlling these actions was difficult because of the maze of channels through which requests for construction were forwarded and approved. After appointment of the base development co-ordinator, these wasteful and uneconomical practices were greatly reduced.

Climate and weather created special problems in site selection and preparation. Buildings flooded during the monsoon rains, requiring extensive dike building and ditch digging to preclude a recurrence. Roads had to be hard-surfaced to be passable during the wet season. Grounds had to be seeded with grass to keep the dust down during the dry season.

Heavy-duty construction equipment itself had to be specially prepared to withstand the dust, mud, humidity, and intense heat.

Electrical power was limited in the cities and lacking in the countryside. Generators were installed to provide the vast quantities of current needed for lighting, air-conditioning units, and the electrically powered equipment of a modern hospital. Water was equally limited. Wells were dug or water piped in to furnish the running water needed for bathing, laundry, sterilization of equipment, and operation of flush toilets. Equipment was installed to make the water potable.

Through the concerted effort of contractors, the Corps of Engineers, and medical personnel, these handicaps were overcome and a series of superb hospitals capable of providing the finest care in every branch of medicine and surgery was established in Vietnam. After returning from Vietnam in 1968, General Collins commented, "Our hospitals in Vietnam are not evacuation hospitals, surgical hospitals, or field hospitals. They are more than that and consequently require sophisticated equipment . . . . We are all interested in providing the best care possible. At present we have some items of equipment in Vietnam that equal what you have at Walter Reed."

Special Units

MUST-equipped surgical hospitals were operated for several years in Vietnam with mixed success. These units consisted of three basic elements, each of which could be airlifted and dispatched by truck or helicopter. The expandable surgical element was a self-contained, rigid-panel shelter with accordion sides. The air-inflatable ward element was a double-walled fabric shelter providing a free-space area for ward facilities. The utility element or power package contained a multifuel gas turbine engine which supplied electric power for air-conditioning, refrigeration, air heating and circulation, water heating and pumping, air pressure for the inflatable elements, and compressed air or suction. In addition, other expandables were used for central materiel supply, laboratory, X-ray, pharmacy, dental, and kitchen facilities.

By 20 October 1966, personnel and MUST equipment of the 45th Surgical Hospital had all arrived in-country. Work was begun on ground preparation and construction of quarters and a mess a few miles west of Tay Ninh. The utility packs and operating room and central materiel expandables had been moved next to the site when it was hit by mortars on 4 November and its commander, Major Gary P. Wratten, MC, was killed.

Two days later the hospital was ordered to become operational as soon as possible to support Operation ATTLEBORO, then in progress northeast of Tay Ninh. An emergency surgical capability and a 20-

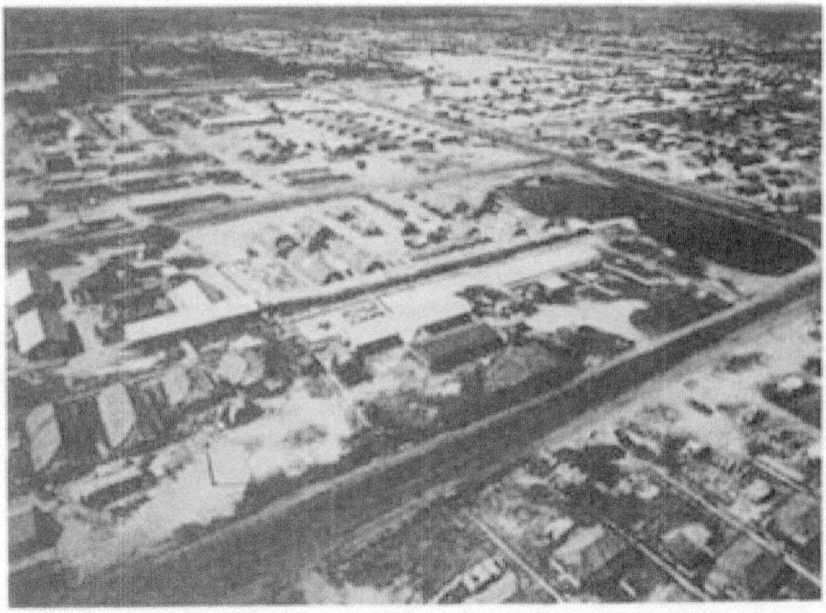

45TH SURGICAL HOSPITAL AT TAY NINH, 1967

patient holding capacity was completed on 8 November. The rest of the hospital was ready to open on 11 November when three more mortar attacks delayed operations until 13 November, when the hospital received its first casualties.

Lieutenant Colonel (later Colonel) Thomas G. Nelson, MC, MUST professional consultant to The Surgeon General, reported in 1967 that, during the early period of its operation, the 45th Surgical Hospital operated as a true forward surgical hospital; that is, patients were not held for followup surgery or prolonged treatment.

Commenting on the relationship between helicopter evacuation and the employment of a forward surgical hospital, he continued:

> As was true of other hospitals in Vietnam, patients were moved directly from the battlefield either to a clearing station or a nearby hospital . . . . Most patients arrived at the hospital within 10 minutes of pickup, and some of these were in such critical condition, usually from internal bleeding or respiratory problems, that further evacuation even by helicopter would likely have been fatal . . . .
>
> Patients were moved from the helicopter pad directly into the preoperative and resuscitation shelter where they were met by the surgical team on-call and the registrar section to initiate resuscitation and medical records. Patients were nearly always admitted in groups of from three to ten, and surgical priorities were established as blood administration and other stabilizing measures were employed and X-ray and laboratory determinations obtained.

The performance of the 45th Surgical Hospital led to the accelerated deployment of MUST equipment for three additional surgical hospitals in 1967: the 3d, 18th, and 22d. In 1968, the 95th Evacuation Hospital was temporarily supplemented with some MUST equipment until the construction of a fixed facility was completed. The 2d Surgical Hospital arrived in Vietnam in 1965 and had a long history of distinguished service before becoming the last unit to be equipped with MUST in January 1969. Meanwhile the Marine Corps was also using MUST equipment.

All medical facilities were vulnerable to enemy attack. On 4 and 11 November 1966, the 45th Surgical Hospital was subjected to mortar attacks. The 3d Surgical Hospital underwent a 15-minute mortar barrage on 24 July 1967, with direct hits on the bachelor officers' quarters and the MUST maintenance hut. Near misses caused extensive damage to practically all inflatable elements. No patients were wounded, although 18 members of the hospital staff received minor wounds. During 1968, the 3d Surgical Hospital underwent 13 attacks which resulted in damage to the hospital area. On 5 and 6 March the hospital suffered extensive damage from mortar and recoilless rifle fire. The headquarters and chapel were completely flattened; the dental clinic, X-ray, laboratory, medical library, medical supply building, and nurses' quarters were all damaged. The intensive care ward and postoperative ward were heavily damaged or destroyed. During this 2-day period, no patients were wounded, although three staff members received minor fragment wounds. Repairs were completed quickly and the hospital remained operational throughout.

Until mid-1968, most field-army-level medical facilities, including MUST units, were not mobile. The 45th and 3d Surgical Hospitals remained stationary after the initial emplacement of MUST equipment. Billets, messhalls, and storage areas were constructed to support the units. Revetments were raised around all inflatable MUST components to make them less vulnerable during attacks. Difficulties in relocating the 18th and 22d Surgical Hospitals earlier in 1968 demonstrated the need to retain mobility. Thus, late in 1968, the USARV surgeon instituted a policy that two MUST surgical hospitals would retain all equipment necessary to be completely mobile and that drills would be held frequently to keep hospital personnel trained to displace, move, and emplace their hospitals rapidly. The 2d and 18th Surgical Hospitals were designated as "mobile" MUST's.

While MUST equipment was an important addition to the inventory of Medical Department assets, it was not used in accordance with doctrine. Its "transportable" attribute was not exploited. Because hospitals supported operations from fixed locations, emphasis was placed on the selection of a hospital site in a reasonably secure area. Proximity to tactical operations was a consideration only in the sense that the hospital had to be within reasonable air-evacuation time and distance. Hospitals had to be moved only when major tactical forces shifted to open new areas of operations, such as, for example, the large-scale buildup of U.S. Army forces in I CTZ during 1968. MUST equipment was a link in such hospital relocations. Pending the construction of fixed facilities in new areas, MUST hospitals provided the controlled environment and the other resources needed for high-quality patient care. As air-conditioned fixed hospitals were completed, the need for MUST equipment diminished. In late 1969, the MUST equipment was withdrawn from the 3d, 18th, and 22d Surgical Hospitals, leaving only two hospitals so equipped. The 3d and 18th Surgical Hospitals were re-established in semipermanent facilities and the 22d Surgical Hospital redeployed to the continental United States. The 2d and 45th Hospitals were closed out in 1970.

The convalescent center. During the visit of The Surgeon General, Lieutenant General Leonard D. Heaton, to Vietnam in early November 1965, General Westmoreland strongly recommended that a convalescent center be established in Vietnam as soon as possible. Malaria was increasing among U.S. forces, and too many patients suffering from malaria or hepatitis were being evacuated out of the country because they could not be hospitalized and returned to duty within the USARV 30-day evacuation policy. General Heaton accepted this recommendation and directed that a convalescent center be established.

The 6th Convalescent Center was activated on 29 November 1965, deployed to Vietnam during March and April 1966, and received its first patients on 15 May. The center was located at Cam Ranh Bay, adjacent to the South China Sea. Its mission was to provide convalescent care for medical and surgical patients, including combat wounded. After a year of operation, approximately 7,500 patients had been admitted to the center from all areas of the country. The patient census averaged more than a thousand a month, with malaria constituting 50 to 65 percent of all admissions. Other admissions included hepatitis patients and those requiring longer periods of postoperative care than 30 days. Approximately 96 percent of all admissions were returned to duty—during an average month, the equivalent of one to two battalions.

Prisoner-of-war hospitalization. During 1965, POW (prisoner-of-war) patients captured by U.S. forces were treated in U.S. medical facilities in the area where they were apprehended. Because of an increase in the number of prisoners, this policy was changed in early 1966. Special medical facilities for the care of prisoners of war, operated by two clearing companies, were constructed at Long Binh and Phu Thanh (near Qui Nhon). Initial major surgery and postoperative care continued to be provided by an Army hospital before the POW patient was moved to a clearing facility. This system created a number of problems. It reduced the number of beds available for U.S. soldiers, mixed prisoners of war with U.S. patients, and required a large number of guards. To alleviate these problems, both clearing facilities were expanded by semipermanent construction into 250-bed hospitals with complete surgical resources.

During 1968, the POW patient load increased from an average of 250 to approximately 400. After several Reserve and National Guard hospitals arrived in October, the 74th Field Hospital assumed the POW mission of the 50th Clearing Company at Long Binh, and the 311th Field Hospital replaced the 542d Clearing Company at Phu Thanh.

During the first half of 1969, the patient load remained fairly constant. Average length of stay for wounded POW patients was 4 to 5 months, and each hospital had a 70- to 80-percent average bed occupancy. After hospitalization, patients were transferred to POW compounds operated by the Vietnamese Army. Upon the redeployment of the reserve hospitals to CONUS during the second half of 1969, the POW hospital mission was reassigned to the 17th Field Hospital and the 24th Evacuation Hospital. A decrease in combat activity reduced the average patient load in each hospital to approximately 100. Because the ARVN (Army Republic of Vietnam) had the largest POW medical workload and the ultimate responsibility for the prisoners' continued confinement, USARV proposed that ARVN administer the entire POW hospitalization program. U.S. Army hospitals would continue to accept and treat prisoners of war captured in their respective geographic areas until their medical condition permitted transfer to an ARVN hospital. In addition, the United States agreed to assist ARVN in reducing the reconstructive and rehabilitative surgical backlog of patients in ARVN hospitals. This concept was implemented in September 1969.

Offshore Support

The patient evacuation policy for Vietnam was established as a 15-day minimum or a 30-day optimum. Under this policy, it was possible to return to duty in Vietnam nearly 40 percent of those injured through hostile action and 70 percent of other surgical patients.

Out-of-country evacuation was by aircraft to Clark Air Force Base in the Philippines; from there evacuees were subsequently routed either to the continental United States, to Tripler General Hospital in Hawaii, to the U.S. Army Hospital, Ryukyu Islands, or to Japan. In the summer of 1966, direct evacuation by jet aircraft of patients from Vietnam to the continental United States via one stop in Japan was inaugurated.

Patients received in the continental United States were mostly accommodated in general hospitals nearest their homes, but some were regulated to class I hospitals even nearer their homes when these hospitals had beds available and the professional capability of treating their injuries.

As the entire Republic of Vietnam had been designated a combat zone, fixed hospitals that give long-term care to patients and are normally found in a communications zone were not present. If all the injured or sick who could not be returned to duty in Vietnam within the established 15- to 30-day evacuation policy had been evacuated to the continental United States, it would have created a great drain of experienced manpower from the combat zone. To give this fixed-bed capability, the equivalent of about 3½ general hospitals were established in Japan to receive and care for patients who could be expected to return to duty within 60 days.

Evacuation

In-Country

Highly mobile and widely deployed forces must have a highly mobile and flexible medical evacuation system immediately responsive to their needs. The helicopter ambulance provided this flexibility and responsiveness in Vietnam. At the peak of combat operations in 1968, aeromedical support was provided by 116 air ambulances. These helicopters could transport six to nine patients at a time, depending upon the number of litter cases. Medical evacuation flights averaged only about 35 minutes each, a feat which often meant the difference between life and death for hundreds of patients. The more seriously wounded usually reached a hospital within 1 to 2 hours after they were injured. Of the wounded who reached medical facilities, about 97.5 percent survived.

The helicopter brought modern medical capabilities closer to the frontline than ever before. Furthermore, combined with a medical radio network, the helicopter provided greater flexibility in regulating patients. Preliminary evaluation of the injury and the condition of the patient was made while in flight, and the use of the radio network permitted redirecting the patient to the nearest hospital suited to his needs. If a hospital developed a surgical backlog, the combination of helicopter and radio facilitated regulating patients according to available operating facilities, rather than available beds. This combination was the core of the Army medical management system in Vietnam.

The buildup of air ambulance units. The buildup of air ambulance units paralleled the commitment of U.S. combat forces to Vietnam. The first air ambulance unit sent to Vietnam, the 57th Medical Detachment (Helicopter Ambulance), later nicknamed "The Originals," arrived in 1962 to support the 8th Field Hospital at Nha Trang. The unit was authorized five HU–1A aircraft, which were replaced by an improved model, the "B" version, in March 1963. Initially, two aircraft were stationed at Qui Nhon and three in Nha Trang. As fighting increased around Saigon and in the Delta, the helicopters were shifted from place to place in response. The 82d Medical Detachment (Helicopter Ambulance) became operational in IV CTZ (the Delta), in November 1964.

The buildup of units continued at an accelerated pace in 1965. The 283d Medical Detachment (Air Ambulance) arrived in August 1965, followed by the 498th Medical Company (Air Ambulance) in September. The 254th Medical Detachment (Air Ambulance) arrived in Vietnam before the end of the year but did not become operational until February 1966 because a backlog at the port delayed the arrival of the unit's equipment. The four detachments, each authorized six helicopters under a new table of organization and equipment, supported III and IV CTZ's. The 498th Medical Company, which was authorized 25 aircraft, supported II CTZ.

During 1967, the 45th Medical Company (Air Ambulance) and four additional air ambulance detachments arrived in Vietnam. The units were shifted from location to location to provide the most effective area coverage in response to tactical operations. In 1968, four additional detachments were sent to Vietnam, completing the buildup of aeromedical evacuation units. One unit, the 50th Medical Detachment, which was assigned to the 101st Airborne Division in mid-1968, became the nucleus of the division's air ambulance platoon. By 1969, there were 116 field-army-level helicopter ambulances in Vietnam. These were assigned to two companies and 11 separate detachments. (*Map 3*)

Air Force aeromedical evacuation support. The Army and the U.S. Air Force evacuation systems complemented each other, each carefully continuing the movement of wounded or sick until they reached a final-destination medical facility.

Based on experience gained in World War II and the Korean War, the U.S. Air Force initially used returning assault or cargo aircraft for casualty evacuation. The system worked well during the early stages of the Vietnam War, because the number of sick and wounded was relatively low. As troop strength increased and combat operations became more intense, the system grew progressively less satisfactory. The requirements for evacuation often coincided with the most urgent needs for resupply, although not always at the same location.

The old system was therefore abandoned in favor of a new one in which aircraft were regularly used specifically for evacuation purposes. The 903d Aeromedical Evacuation Squadron scheduled the first regular in-country evacuation flights in 1967. By late 1969, the number of regular scheduled flights had increased to 188. The assault aircraft initially used for aeromedical evacuation were supplemented, in early 1968, by C-118 cargo aircraft specifically modified for evacuation missions. The average

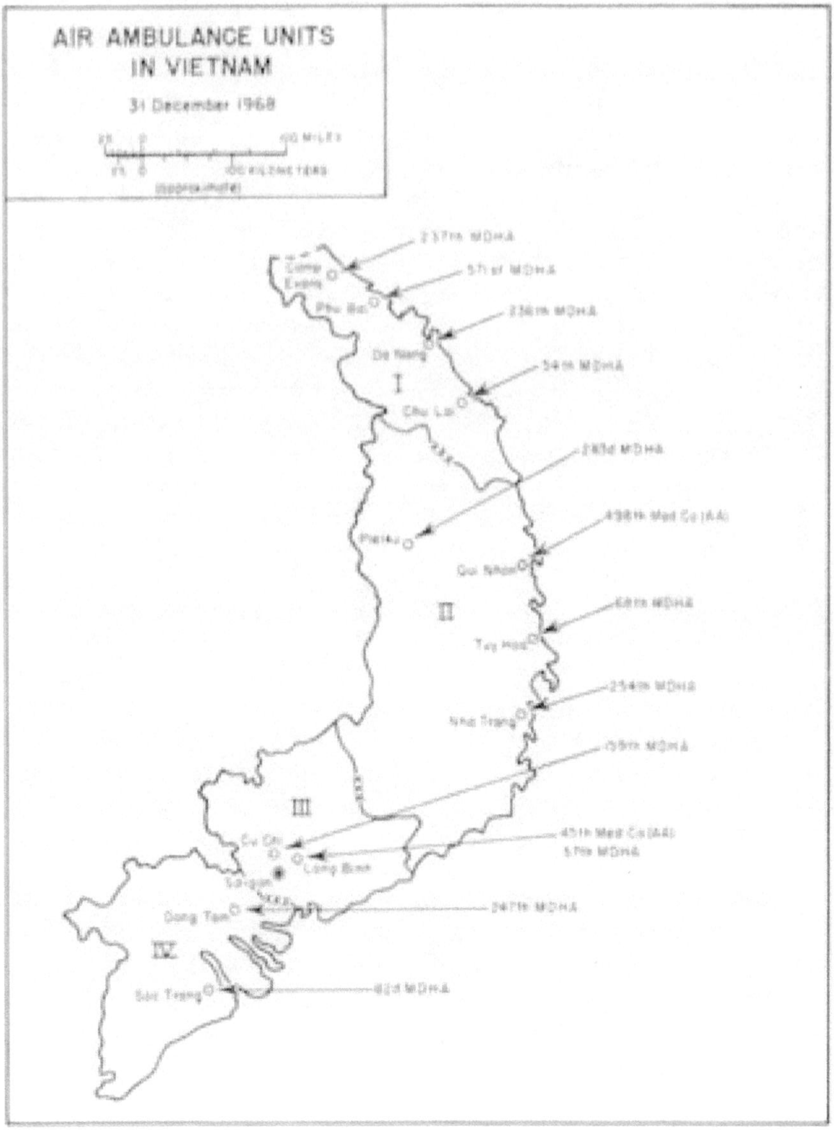

Map 3

number of patients moved increased from 5,813 per month between July 1967 and January 1968, to 9,098 from March to June 1968. During the Tet Offensive in February 1968, more than 10,000 patients were evacuated by the Air Force.

"Dust-off." Those Army medical evacuation helicopter units not organic to divisions came to be called Dust-off, after the radio call sign of

the most famous of the early pilots, Major Charles L. Kelly, MSC, who was killed in action on 1 July 1964. Several scores of these flying "medics" flew their unarmed helicopters into hostile areas, risking their own lives to save those of others. In a 2-year period, 39 crew members were killed and 210 wounded in aeromedical evacuation missions.

The combination of the helicopter ambulance and a medical radio network was the basis of the effective medical regulating system that evolved in Vietnam. During the first phase of U.S. troop commitment to Vietnam in early 1965, there was only one hospital in support of each CTZ and therefore no alternative to the destination of a casualty. As the number of hospitals and the number of casualties increased, however, the need for a regulating system became imperative. The first system in the III and IV CTZ's was set up with Air Force Radar Tan Son Nhut, Paris control. Dust-off helicopters inbound called Paris control which had a direct-line field telephone "hot line" to the MRO (medical regulating office) and the 3d Field Hospital. The three major treatment facilities available were the 3d Field Hospital, the 93d Evacuation Hospital, and the 3d Surgical Hospital, the last named then located at Bien Hoa. The MRO confirmed or changed the destination chosen by the pilot as the medical situation indicated.

After Headquarters, 44th Medical Brigade, arrived in Vietnam in 1966, the brigade MRO became responsible for all in-country regulating of patients. Medical groups controlled the movement of patients from tactical areas to hospitals within their own group areas. Further movement of patients from one group area to another was co-ordinated by medical group MRO's with the brigade MRO, who maintained over-all control to insure proper usage of all medical facilities.

Telephone communications were abysmally poor and radio communications not much better during this period. When heavy fighting produced a large number of casualties and medical regulating was most urgently needed, operational radio traffic was also heaviest. Moreover, since short-range radios were used, requests for evacuation had to be routed from divisional medical battalions to backup hospitals by way of the Dust-off radio network or through the supporting field army medical group. This cumbersome method caused delays and sometimes resulted in garbled transmissions.

On an experimental basis, the 55th Medical Group at Qui Nhon borrowed single-sideband long-range radios from the 498th Medical Company (Air Ambulance). Originally placed in the air ambulance company for long-range transmissions to its aircraft on evacuation missions, these radios had been little used because of the relatively short distance of most flights and the extensive maintenance they required. Their use for medical regulating proved highly successful, and an additional 54 sets were ultimately acquired to expand the communications network throughout the medical brigade.

Medical regulating started on the battlefield. Medical groups placed regulators (senior noncommissioned officers) in areas of troop concentration or at the site of a combat operation. In co-operation with the local medical unit, the regulator radioed requests for evacuation to the supporting Dust-off unit. The transmission was monitored by the MRO at his medical group headquarters.

In the absence of a field medical regulator, a request for air evacuation was normally made by the medical aidman at the site of the casualty. The request, which included such information as the number of patients by type, the exact location by map grid co-ordinates, data on enemy movements, and the radio frequency of the requesting unit, was transmitted over the Dust-off radio network to the supporting air ambulance unit. Frequently the call was received by an air ambulance already in flight which could be diverted from a less urgent mission. If not, a standby crew at a field site or at the unit headquarters scrambled to make the pickup.

After proper identification of the ground force with the casualty, the Dust-off helicopter generally made a high-speed or tight-circle approach into the area. Time spent on the ground in a normal operation was usually between 30 seconds and 1 minute, depending on the number of casualties. The casualty was given emergency treatment by the medical aidman on board as soon as the aircraft was out of the combat area.

The patient was flown directly to the medical treatment facility best able to give the care required. This might or might not be the one nearest the site of injury. The decision as to the proper destination hospital was based on several factors. Distance was less important than time; the objective was to reduce the time between injury and definitive treatment to the minimum. Information based on the preliminary in-flight evaluation of the injury and the condition of the patient, knowledge of existing surgical backlogs, and the over-all casualty situation were other considerations. If the aircraft commander questioned the destination selected by the medical regulator because of his knowledge of the patient's condition, a physician was consulted by radio while the patient was still in transit before the decision became final. The inbound medical aircraft commander informed the receiving hospital by radio of his estimated time of arrival, the nature of the casualties on board, and any special reception arrangements that might be required. Thus, the receiving hospital was able to have everything in order to receive casualties and begin definitive surgical care.

Helicopter evacuation techniques and requirements varied by geographic area, type of combat operation, and type of equipment available, and changed from year to year as experience modified and refined procedures. Since the air ambulance was unarmed, gunship support was requested if the ground reported contact with the enemy in the vicinity of the pickup site, or if the rescue was a hoist operation.

In "hot" areas, the crew of the evacuation aircraft consisted of a pilot, copilot, crew chief, medical aidman, and a man armed with an automatic rifle. In quieter areas, the rifleman was left behind in favor of increased patient capacity. On hoist operations in mountainous and jungle terrain, before the more powerful "H" model aircraft was introduced, the crew consisted only of a pilot, copilot, and hoist operator. On these missions, fuel load was also generally reduced in favor of greater lift capability. Night missions were quite common, often comprising 15 to 20 percent of the total missions in some areas.

Helicopter rescue operations were aided by new equipment designed especially for use in jungle terrain or in combat areas where it was too dangerous for a helicopter to land. The hoist consisted of a winch and cable on a boom which was moved out from the aircraft when it arrived over the rescue site. At the end of the cable was a ring and hook to which a Stokes litter, rigid litter, or forest penetrator could be attached. The cable could be lowered at the rate of 150 feet per minute and retracted at the rate of 120 feet per minute. The forest penetrator, a spring-loaded device which could penetrate dense foliage, opened to provide seats on which a casualty could be strapped. It was preferred over the litter by the crews for hoist rescues because it was less likely to become entangled in the trees.

Hoist operations significantly increased the danger for Dust-off crews. Hovering above the jungle or a mountain side as it lowered its cable, the helicopter became a "sitting duck" for enemy troops in the area. In 1968, 35 aircraft were hit by hostile fire while on hoist missions. The number increased to 39 in 1969. Nonetheless, the hoist was used extensively and to great advantage in Vietnam. Its use permitted the rescue of 1,735 casualties in 1968 and 2,516 casualties in 1969, who otherwise could not have been retrieved.

The primary mission of the Army helicopter ambulance was the in-country aeromedical evacuation of patients. The number of patients evacuated by aeromedical evacuation helicopters rose from 13,004 in 1965, to 67,910 in 1966, to 85,804 in 1967, and peaked at 206,229 in 1969. These figures included members of the ARVN, Vietnamese civilians, and Free World forces as well as U.S. patients. Each time a patient was moved by helicopter, the move was entered in the tally. Thus, if a patient was taken to a surgical hospital by helicopter and later transported from there to an evacuation hospital by helicopter, this would count as two patients evacuated. Army air ambulances completed more

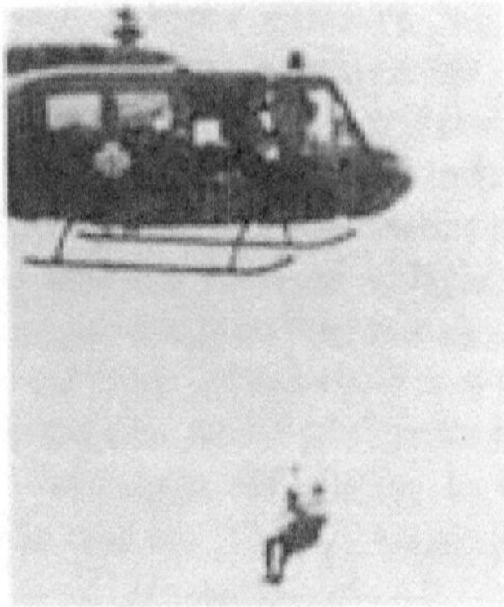

USE OF HOIST IN VIETNAM, 1968

than 104,112 aeromedical evacuation missions while flying approximately 78,652 combat hours in 1969.

In addition to this primary mission, Army helicopters were also used to transport professional personnel, medical supplies, and blood to medical facilities. Supplemented by scheduled Air Force flights, and from time to time by larger helicopters, they were also used to transport patients between hospitals for consultations or to free beds in areas where increased casualties were anticipated.

Out-of-Country

The Air Force provided all out-of-country aeromedical evacuation. Initially, out-of-country medical regulating was controlled at the FEJMRO (Far East Medical Regulating Office) at Camp Zama, Japan, through a representative functioning at the Office of the Surgeon, USMACV. To handle the increased volume of traffic, a branch of the FEJMRO was established in Vietnam and Major (later Lieutenant Colonel) Robert M. Latham, MSC, reported as Chief, FEJMRO (USMACV), in July 1966. FEJMRO allotted bed space in hospitals in the Pacific area for FEJMRO (USMACV) use, and issued "bed credits" on a 24-hour basis. This information was relayed to Vietnam via Clark Air Force Base in the Philippines because communications between Japan and Vietnam were chronically poor. Late in 1966, a direct system for transmitting information between the two offices was adopted.

The procedures for regulating out-of-country evacuations were further improved in November 1967. Under these new procedures, medical group regulating officers submitted consolidated requests for evacuation to the medical brigade MRO who then sent a single request to FEJMRO (USMACV). In turn, information concerning destination hospitals was sent back down the line. The new system enabled hospitals in Vietnam to follow up on patients and permitted medical facilities to close out clinical records. It also provided information more promptly on the total number of evacuees to casualty staging facilities, the Military Airlift Command, and offshore hospitals. Routine calls were handled within a 36-hour period, and urgent evacuation requests were processed within an hour if an aircraft was available.

Since substantial U.S. forces were committed to Vietnam in 1965, the relative continuity of combat was as much a factor in building up patient loads as was the severity of fighting. Under such conditions, patient evacuation was therefore accelerated to provide for contingencies. The 9th Aeromedical Evacuation Squadron, for example, increased its flight schedule from two weekly departures from Tan Son Nhut to daily flights with additional sites for departure at Da Nang and Qui Nhon. The number of evacuations out-of-country increased from 10,164 in 1965 to 35,916 in 1969. (*Table 8*)

TABLE 8.—TOTAL NUMBER OF PATIENTS EVACUATED FROM VIETNAM, U.S. ARMY, BY MONTH, 1965–69

Month	1965	1966	1967	1968	1969
January	164	832	1, 469	2, 417	3, 224
February	227	1, 330	1, 851	3, 576	3, 099
March	226	1, 062	2, 178	2, 471	4, 166
April	252	853	1, 780	2, 782	3, 210
May	300	1, 298	2, 367	3, 952	4, 334
June	480	1, 256	2, 072	2, 701	3, 951
July	471	766	1, 595	2, 569	2, 879
August	821	957	1, 521	2, 700	3, 308
September	999	942	1, 431	3, 401	2, 187
October	1, 978	983	1, 851	2, 856	1, 890
November	2, 361	1, 331	2, 435	2, 790	1, 789
December	1, 885	996	2, 152	3, 176	1, 879
Total	10, 164	12, 606	22, 702	35, 391	35, 916

Source: Army Medical Service Activities Report, MACV, 1965; Army Medical Service Activities Reports, 44th Medical Brigade, 1966, 1967, 1968, 1969.

Initially, out-of-country evacuation was by aircraft to Clark Air Force Base; from there evacuees were routed either to the continental United States; to Tripler General Hospital in Hawaii, to the U.S. Army Hospital, Ryukyu Islands, or to Japan. In the summer of 1966, to reduce the drain of experienced manpower from the combat zone, the equivalent of about 3½ general hospitals was established in Japan to receive and care for patients who could be returned to duty within a 60-day period. C–141 Starlifter jets, which were used to transport troops to Vietnam, were quickly reconfigured to evacuate patients to Japan. The C–141 could carry 80 litter, 121 ambulatory, or a combination of 36 litter and 54 ambulatory patients. After a 6-hour flight to Japan where those patients to be retained disembarked, patients bound for the continental United States boarded and the aircraft continued either to Andrews Air Force Base, Washington, D.C. (18 hours via Elmendorf Air Force Base, Alaska) or to Travis Air Force Base, Calif., by a direct 10-hour flight.

Throughout the chain of evacuation, the well-being of the patient was of overriding concern. At all points along the chain, a qualified flight surgeon was on hand to determine if the evacuation should be continued. If necessary, a physician accompanied a severely wounded or critically ill patient. At all times, the finest medical care was given to the wounded or sick soldier as he progressed through the aeromedical evacuation system.

Reduction and Reorganization

The de-escalation of combat activities in Vietnam during 1969 and 1970 was paralleled by a reduction in the number of hospitals and air ambulance units. During 1969, three Reserve hospitals returned to the continental United States. The 7th and 22d Surgical Hospitals and the 29th and 36th Evacuation Hospitals were inactivated. The number of beds in operation decreased from 5,189 to 3,473 by the end of the year. During 1970, the 8th Field, the 2d Surgical, the 45th Surgical, and the 12th Evacuation Hospitals were redeployed or inactivated. (*Map 4*) The 254th Medical Detachment (Helicopter Ambulance) was inactivated in November.

A new structure for administering the medical units still in-country was authorized. Early in 1970, outlying dispensaries and clinics were placed under the command and control of the hospital in the closest geographic proximity. This change resulted in the inactivation of the headquarters elements of two medical battalions. The two medical battalions in-country were reorganized and given command and control of all medical evacuation helicopter, field ambulance, and bus ambulance resources. One medical evacuation battalion was assigned to each of the two medical groups that remained in Vietnam.

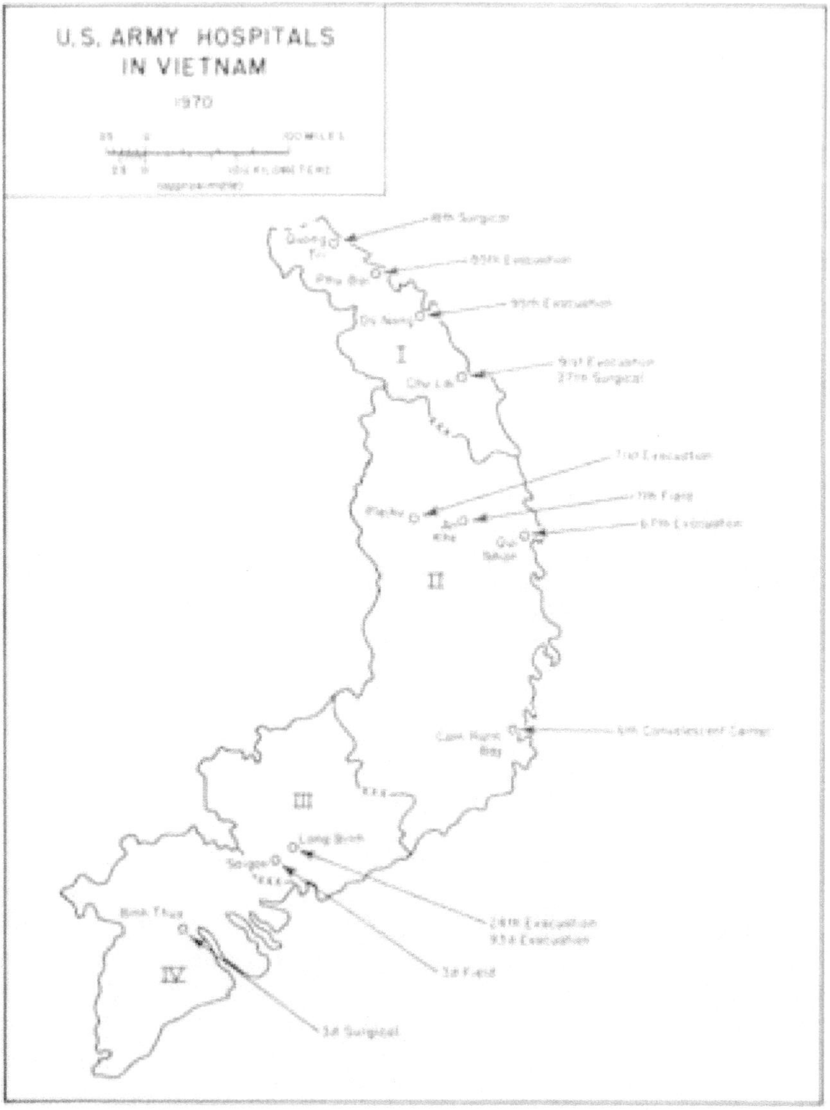
U.S. ARMY HOSPITALS
IN VIETNAM
1970
Da Nang
I
Chu Lai
II
III
Long Binh
Saigon
IV

Map 4

CHAPTER V
Medical Supply

Realignment of Medical Supply Activities

Medical Materiel Management in Overseas Commands: 1962–66

After the reorganization of the Department of the Army headquarters in 1962, supply activities in overseas commands were consolidated within supply agencies organized on a functional basis. Medical supply was incorporated within the functional systems although in each instance the command surgeon objected to the change, contending that there would be a serious deterioration in support to medical facilities and medical units.

Under the new system, supply management activities for USARPAC were centralized at the Inventory Control Point in Hawaii. The Inventory Control Point was responsible for controlling of all requisitioning of supplies within the command and for the centralized maintenance of records on the status of supplies for the Eighth U.S. Army in Korea as well as for U.S. Army units in Japan, Hawaii, and Okinawa.

Medical Materiel Support of the Troop Buildup

The disadvantages in treating medical materiel as just another category of supply items were quickly and unequivocally exposed in 1965 when Army medical materiel units were faced with an expanded support mission—the buildup of U.S. Army troops in Vietnam. One of the most significant supply problems at the onset of the buildup was a lack of adequate medical supply personnel in the theater as well as the lack of continuity in key positions resulting from the 12-month Vietnam tour of duty.

The 8th Field Hospital at Nha Trang was responsible for medical supply distribution to the medical units in Vietnam. This unit was augmented by a small staff which was not adequate to provide the necessary control over the tremendous requirements being generated practically overnight. This situation was compounded by the protracted delay in deployment of the 32d (Field Army) Medical Depot which, although "ready" in July 1965, was not deployed until late October. One supply detachment had been deployed in July and another shortly thereafter, but these detachments did not have a sufficient depth to manage supply activities in a theater of operations the size of Vietnam.

With the escalation of U.S. efforts in Vietnam, greater dependence was placed upon the Ryukyu Islands as the offshore base to support units in Vietnam. A supply detachment was deployed to Okinawa in August, and in November 1965, the 70th Medical Depot was deployed to augment and expand the operation of the medical depot in Okinawa.

The Surgeon General, handicapped by insufficient strength and control of medical supply, co-ordinated with CINCPAC to establish a system of automatic shipments of medical materiel to Vietnam. These shipments, initiated in July 1965, were based upon schedules developed to support forces which were deployed from the continental United States to Vietnam. The materiel shipped consisted primarily of medical resupply sets and later, after their development, included optical resupply sets. The automatic supply support system continued for a period of approximately 10 months, with peakloads of resupply occurring from November 1965 through January 1966. This system, although only a temporary measure, was not so successful as anticipated. Delays in shipment from CONUS ports and in off-loading procedures at Vietnam facilities and the splitting of the medical resupply sets into various shipments on board vessels were the major difficulties experienced.

Investigation of Malfunctions in the Medical Supply System

By mid-1965, the Army medical materiel supply system was close to a complete breakdown because of the lack of qualified medical logistics personnel in Vietnam, the shortcomings of the medical resupply system related previously, and the inability of a centralized supply management activity in Hawaii to meet the medical materiel demands in Vietnam. In November 1965, the Vice Chief of Staff directed The Surgeon General to investigate and recommend appropriate measures to resolve these difficulties and end the shortages occurring in Vietnam and other subordinate commands within USARPAC. A representative of The Surgeon General investigated and found that the Inventory Control Point, USARPAC, could not provide pertinent data on the medical supply situation within USARPAC. Consequently, requisitioning objectives were being computed without the full knowledge of subordinate command conditions, environment, or professional requirements. In fact, to insure adequacy of objectives, subordinate commands had to review their records constantly and thus engage in duplication of effort. The investigation revealed that the Inventory Control Point provided little assistance to the subordinate commands or to the surgeons who were responsible for the health of troops in those subordinate commands. The report indicated that the medical commodity group was not large enough to require management within a centralized and functionalized system; however, it was important enough to require extraordinary management under the direction of the subordinate command surgeons to support peacetime and wartime operations.

The status of medical supply in each of the subordinate commands disclosed large numbers of medical items with zero balances (complete lack of stock). This situation necessitated submitting large numbers of high priority requisitions to CONUS to obtain vitally needed stocks rapidly.

The report further indicated that the rapid buildup of troop strength in Vietnam had placed a serious drain on available medical materiel stocks in the DSA (Defense Supply Agency) system. For example, of the 6,000 to 7,000 medical items on hand, DSA was out of stock on about 1,500 items and these were articles needed in the field to administer first aid. Delays in shipments and out-of-stock conditions became more serious as the buildup progressed. In Okinawa, the offshore support base, for example, zero balances rose from 16 percent in December 1964, to 28 percent in March 1965. Unfortunately, The Surgeon General was not fully informed of the deficiencies until complaints were received from Vietnam and other USARPAC areas.

While the inadequacies and malfunctioning of the supply system were being investigated, a concept study advocating a bold, new approach to the problem of the administrative support of a theater army, entitled "TASTA-70 (The Administrative Support-Theater Army 1965–70)," was under study in the Office of the Chief of Staff. Commenting on the study, The Surgeon General recommended that the Army Medical Department be given control over medical depots and medical inventory control activities. Approved by the Chief of Staff, The Surgeon General's recommendation was incorporated in the TASTA-70 concept and provided the basis for the realignment of medical supply activities under the command surgeons in overseas commands which began in the summer of 1966.

The Surgeon General's Plan

During the summer of 1966, the medical supply system supporting military activities in Vietnam was realigned by shifting the responsibility for determining requisition objectives for stocked medical items and for ordering replenishment supplies from the Inventory Control Point to the U.S. Army Medical Depot in the Ryukyu Islands. This depot, in turn, ordered replenishment supplies directly from the Defense Personnel Support Center through the USAMMA (U.S. Army Medical Materiel Agency), Phoenixville, Pa.

The effect of this realignment was the routing of all requisitions for medical materiel from subordinate commands within USARPAC to the USAMMA, where the order was recorded and reviewed before it was transmitted to the Defense Personnel Support Center, the agency of the Defense Supply Agency which handled medical materiel. Thus, USAMMA was able to maintain control and "followup" on each requisition to insure that the requesting agency was kept fully informed on the status of its order and, when necessary, to expedite the delivery of urgently needed items. USAMMA also prepared and maintained a catalog of nonstandard items for the Pacific area. This catalog facilitated requisitioning of items that were not in the standard supply system and permitted the accumulation of data on worldwide usage of nonstandard items to determine the need for type classification actions.

In 1967, the medical supply section within USARPAC, the Materiel Management Agency, was transferred to the Chief Surgeon, USARPAC, thus completing the shift of all medical supply activities in the Pacific command to medical channels. After this transfer, the Chief Surgeon, USARPAC, was responsible for directing all medical supply functions within the command. In each subordinate command, medical supply responsibilities were assigned to medical commanders and surgeons; for example, in Vietnam, the Surgeon, USARV, was responsible for medical supply functions to include the operations of the 32d Medical Depot, and the operation of the U.S. Army Medical Depot, Ryukyu Islands, was a responsibility of the U.S. Army Medical Center, Ryukyu Islands. Similarly, the U.S. Army Medical Command, Japan, directed the functions of the 504th Medical Depot; the 6th Medical Depot in Korea was assigned as a function of the Surgeon, Eighth U.S. Army; and medical supply activities in Hawaii were incorporated within the structure of Tripler Army Medical Center.

The Depot System

As a result of this assignment of medical materiel mangement the Okinawa depot expanded in size and responsibilities. The depot ultimately supported U.S. Army units in Vietnam and Thailand; the Armed Forces of Vietnam, Thailand, and Laos; and AID (Agency for International Development) activities in Southeast Asia, while also supplying military customers on the Ryukyu Islands. The amount of depot sales to customers rose from $28.5 million in fiscal year 1967 to $64 million in fiscal year 1968 and peaked at $71.5 million in fiscal year 1969. The depot satisfied over 85 percent of the demands for stocked items during fiscal year 1968. The depot also provided optical and medical equipment maintenance support to all areas which it supplied.

In Vietnam, the 32d Medical Depot, which had deployed in October 1965 and which received its medical materiel support from the Okinawa depot, provided medical materiel for units of the U.S. Army and the Armed Forces of Korea, the Philippines, Australia, and New Zealand, operating in Vietnam. During fiscal year 1968, for example, the 32d Medical Depot issued about $30 million of medical materiel in Vietnam and filled more than 85 percent of all requisitions submitted by medical units. Shipments of medical supplies increased from 482 short tons per month in the first quarter of fiscal year 1968 to 932 short tons per month in the third quarter. The depot's functions included the fabrication of single-vision spectacles—in fiscal year 1970 alone the depot produced 170,279 pairs—and the maintenance and repair of medical equipment of supported units throughout Vietnam. The depot operated through five locations (four advance depots and a base depot at Cam Ranh Bay).

Despite chronic shortages of personnel and equipment, the 32d Medical Depot continued to fulfill its mission in a superb manner. By 1970, the medical supply support had reached an operational plateau as medical units and facilities received a routine replenishment of medical supplies. The Army Medical Depot, Ryukyu Islands, also continued to provide replenishment supplies to the Vietnamese Armed Forces, and military assistance supplies for Thailand and Laos forces, and for AID activities in Vietnam, Thailand, and Laos. Medical supplies valued at $71.5 million were distributed through this depot during the fiscal year.

Mechanization of Medical Materiel Recordkeeping

The improvement of medical support in Vietnam was based on the excellent support rendered to the 32d Medical Depot by the U.S. Army Medical Depot, Okinawa, and in-country procedural, organizational, and facility improvement. The depot installed the NCR (National Cash Register Co.) 500 computer system to mechanize stock control and inventory management at the base depot in Cam Ranh Bay and at two advance depots in Long Binh and Qui Nhon in 1967. By 1968, it was apparent that the NCR 500 computers were not adequate to provide the data necessary for decision making, plot supply trends, forecast trouble areas, or program financial inventory data. The depot therefore developed its own programs, borrowed computer time on an IBM (International Business Machines) 360 computer system in Saigon, and produced the information necessary to operate effectively in an environment that was rapidly becoming increasingly management and cost conscious.

By the fall of 1968, the 32d Medical Depot produced the first theater stock status report. The report was developed by converting data from the NCR 500 computer system to cards which were processed in the IBM 360 system. By the spring of 1969, additional advances had been made in the automation of medical materiel recordkeeping. These advances included the preparation of theater excess reports, financial inventory feeder data, due in and due out reconciliation reports, order and shipping time studies, and interdepot redistribution of assets studies. In light of these achievements, plans were made and submitted for comparable support in 1969, and a data automation requirement to automate medical materiel management in Vietnam was approved by the Department of the Army in February 1969.

Transportation and Communication Problems

The reliable transmission of requisitions or supply information was a continuing problem within Vietnam and to a lesser degree between Vietnam and Okinawa. The primary modes of communication were transceiver, mail, and telephone. The transceiver was used between advance depots and the base depot whenever possible and mail was the alternative. Policy changes were sent to the advance depots by transceiver or mail and high-priority requisitions were telephoned to the base depot. To prevent losses of requisitions transceivered between depots, which was not uncommon, batch control techniques were established and proved highly successful.

Transporting supplies within the depot system presented difficulties at times. The road network was poor and often interdicted by the enemy. Under these circumstances, the helicopter was used to pick up supplies from designated supply points and to deliver high-priority requisitions. Bulk quantities of resupply were packed in Conex containers and airlifted by Chinook helicopters.

Improvement of Storage Facilities

Lack of adequate and sufficient storage space for medical supplies was a chronic problem in Vietnam. The acquisition of additional storage space continually lagged behind actual needs. The redistribution of troops compounded matters and storage requirements for medical supplies were frequently overlooked in planning programs. During the early part of the war, there was an acute lack of sufficient covered storage space for the protection of delicate or perishable medical supplies; it was not unusual to find medical supplies being stored in temperatures above 100° F. although boxes were plainly marked not to be stored in temperatures exceeding 80 degrees. Through the vigorous efforts of the 32d Depot, these inadequacies were gradually overcome, and facilities for the proper storage of medical supplies were constructed.

Medical Equipment Maintenance Support

The deployment of medical units and hospitals to Vietnam during 1965 and 1966 precipitated various problems in medical equipment maintenance support. The 32d Medical Depot base platoon general and direct support facility, which was located at Nha Trang, operated out of temporary buildings with inadequate storage and shop space. Hospitals within Vietnam had little or no maintenance capability and were thus dependent upon the base depot for support. Although the 32d Medical Depot had deployed to Vietnam with a prescribed load of repair parts, the supply proved inadequate because of the early approval of many complex and highly specialized items of medical equipment for use in-country. A majority of these items were nonstandard and consequently required nonstandard repair parts which were not included in the original load. During late 1966 and early 1967, the depot incorporated many standard and nonstandard items into a depot maintenance float for direct exchange by units using them; this action made repair parts available to medical facilities within the depot system.

With the establishment of backup maintenance support at the U.S. Army Medical Depot, Okinawa, a number of problems were solved. For example, it was no longer necessary to send 100 MA X-ray tubes to CONUS for repair, a step which involved considerable delay in getting the equipment back into the depot system.

By 1968, tremendous improvements had been made in medical maintenance support and capability. The base depot maintenance section was moved to Cam Ranh Bay and new facilities were programmed for construction. Repair parts management was transferred from maintenance repair personnel to inventory managers, thus enabling the repairmen to devote more time to the actual repair of equipment. In addition, medical equipment assistance teams, composed of highly skilled technicians, responded to the needs of medical facilities for periodic technical assistance and on-site repair.

CHAPTER VI

Division and Brigade Medical Support

Two impressive aspects of medical operations in support of combat units in Vietnam were the versatility of the classic system and the far-reaching modifications of the system that evolved from the Vietnamese experience.

Doctrine prescribed the structure and type of medical support for combat units sent to Vietnam. A medical battalion of four companies, each with three platoons, supported each division. A single medical company supported each separate brigade. The medical platoon of three sections supported units of infantry and tank battalions or armored cavalry squadrons. Under the fluid conditions of warfare in Vietnam, the employment and deployment of combat units determined the utilization of their supporting medical units, and no two medical battalions were used alike. The action accounts that follow are representative of these varied usages.

Usages of Divisional Medical Assets

1st Cavalry Division (Airmobile)

In September 1965, the 1st Cavalry Division (Airmobile), supported by the 15th Medical Battalion (Airmobile), arrived at the Central Highlands bases of Qui Nhon and An Khe lying southeast of Pleiku. In October the North Vietnamese Army began a major operation in the Central Highlands, opening its campaign with an attack on the Plei Me Special Forces camp 25 miles southwest of Pleiku. The 1st Brigade, 1st Cavalry Division (Airmobile), was moved into the area south and west of Pleiku to block any further enemy advance and to stand in readiness as a reaction force. On 27 October, the 1st Cavalry Division (Airmobile) was directed to seek out and destroy the enemy force in western Pleiku province. Thus began the month-long campaign known as the Battle of the Ia Drang Valley. The great effectiveness of the airmobile division was demonstrated in its first combat trial.

The Ia Drang campaign also proved the worth of the airmobile medical support battalion. An innovation, the airmobile medical battalion differed structurally in several ways from the conventional medical battalion. The most important difference was that it included an air ambulance platoon of 12 helicopters and an aircraft maintenance section.

Doctrinally, the division of responsibility between air ambulances organic to a division and Army-level, or Dust-off helicopters, was clear cut. Divisional air ambulances evacuated patients in the division's area of operations from the site of wounding to one of the division's four clearing stations. Dust-off helicopters evacuated patients from the divisional clearing station to an Army hospital. In practice, the line of demarcation was often blurred. During lulls in combat, divisional aircraft flew patients from the clearing station to a hospital, while during peak periods of combat, Army-level helicopters supplemented divisional aircraft and evacuated casualties from the frontline to the divisional clearing station. Occasionally, assault helicopters were used when the medical air evacuation platoon was overtaxed, but Dust-off was preferred because the medical aidman aboard could give emergency treatment and because the patient could be regulated to the hospital best suited to his needs.

In contrast to the usual practice in Vietnam of evacuating a casualty directly from the site of wounding to a hospital by air ambulance, 95 percent of the casualties in the 1st Cavalry Division (Airmobile) were first evacuated to one of the division's clearing stations, because of the size of the division's area of operations. The remaining 5 percent, severely wounded or critically ill patients who could not have survived a stop en route, were evacuated directly to the 45th Surgical Hospital in Tay Ninh or the 2d Surgical Hospital in Lai Khe.

Since there was no difference in flying time from the combat area to the helipad of the clearing station of the 15th Medical Battalion (Airmobile) and that of the 45th Surgical Hospital at Tay Ninh, patients were evacuated to the clearing station. The two units complemented each other. Personnel at the clearing station became adept in the triage of combat casualties and in the techniques—such as administering blood and reducing shock—of stabilizing a seriously wounded patient. Surgeons at the 45th Surgical Hospital, in turn, were freed to devote their full effort to resuscitative surgery without fear that the condition of patients awaiting surgery would deteriorate. The clearing station handled a surprisingly large number of casualties in a short period of time. It also weeded out the slightly wounded and the "sick, lame, and lazy" who would have become the responsibility of the 45th Surgical Hospital had they been evacuated there originally.

25th Infantry Division

In contrast to the relationship between the 15th Medical Battalion (Airmobile) and the 45th Surgical Hospital, casualties from the 25th Infantry Division, which also operated in the Tay Ninh area, were evacuated directly to the 45th Surgical Hospital by Dust-off helicopters which operated from the hospital's helipad. Use of the 25-bed facility adjacent to the 45th Surgical Hospital operated by Company D, 25th Medical Battalion, which supported the 25th Infantry Division, was limited to the care of the patient with a minor illness or a slight wound.

To elaborate further on the contrast between these two methods, the 15th Medical Battalion (Airmobile) operated a clearing station and used the 45th Surgical Hospital in the classic role of a surgical hospital. Company D, 25th Medical Battalion, provided a holding area for patients who could be returned to duty in a few days. Under this arrangement, the 45th Surgical Hospital also served as a clearing station.

The same relationship existed between the remaining companies of the 25th Medical Battalion and the 12th Evacuation Hospital at Chu Lai. The three companies together operated a single 25-bed facility as a holding area. The 12th Evacuation Hospital served as a clearing station as well as an evacuation hospital.

In 1968, the 25th Medical Battalion operated facilities at three locations and treated 75,184 patients. Dust-off helicopters flew 8,159 missions and evacuated more than 20,000 patients. In 1969, the 25th Medical Battalion treated more than 58,000 patients. That same year, Dust-off aircraft flew approximately 7,000 missions and evacuated about 14,000 patients.

326th Medical Battalion

During its service in Vietnam, the 326th Medical Battalion was converted from an airborne to an airmobile unit. It lost some men and ground vehicles and acquired an air ambulance platoon which became known as "Eagle Dust-off." This conversion paralleled the conversion of the 101st Airborne Division to the 101st Air Cavalry Division to the 101st Airborne Division (Airmobile). Even so, the battalion still did not match the table of organization for an airmobile medical battalion. Instead, it operated under a modified table of organization.

To insure adequate medical support for the 101st Airborne Division (Airmobile) which operated primarily in the vicinity of Hue and Phu Bai, except for its 3d Brigade which was retained in the critical Saigon area, all elements of the 326th Medical Battalion were monitored and evaluated continually. As a result of this surveillance, changes were made from time to time to improve the unit's performance. For example, four litter bearers, one from each medical company, were deleted in exchange for four preventive medicine specialists who were added to the staff of the division surgeon.

Mobile Riverine Force

The Mobile Riverine Force, created in 1967, was composed of the 2d Brigade, 9th Infantry Division, and two Navy river assault squadrons of 50 boats each. The force, designed to deny the extensive river and canal complex of the Mekong Delta to the enemy, was wholly independent of fixed support bases and operated entirely afloat. Company D, 9th Medical Battalion, supported the Mobile Riverine Force in a highly unorthodox manner. Shortly after Company D arrived at the Dong Tam base in early 1968, it established a medical facility in a converted armored troop carrier to provide more effective medical support for riverine operations. Later this facility, the only Army medical facility in Vietnam based in a Navy ship, was moved to a barracks ship, the U.S.S. *Colleton*. After the arrival of Company A, 9th Medical Battalion, at Dong Tam in August 1968, Company D established a 37-bed facility for medical cases aboard the U.S.S. *Nueces*, thus freeing the unit on the *Colleton* for care of surgical patients. When the U.S.S. *Mercer* replaced the *Colleton* a few months later, the medical and surgical units were united aboard the *Nueces*. The rear section of the aid station of Company D was maintained in these ships at the base anchorage.

On tactical operations, Navy armored troop carriers, preceded by minesweeping craft and escorted by armored boats, transported the soldiers along the vast network of waterways in the Delta. The units debarked upon reaching the area of operations or upon contact with the enemy.

Small, specially designed craft with an aid station aboard, called aid boats, accompanied the troop boats into combat. A physician, attached to Company D during these riverine operations, went forward on an aid boat with the combat units. The aid boats functioned at night when most combat in the Delta took place. Casualties were evacuated to the ship-based rear aid station at the base anchorage by aid boats or by helicopters permanently assigned to the Mobile Riverine Force, at first by the Army and later by the Navy.

The primary medical problem in riverine operations was "immersion foot," which was minimized by alternating units in combat every 2 or 3 days. While the fresh troops sustained the attack, those units relieved were allowed to "dry out" and refit.

Riverine operations brought extensive modifications in the use of personnel and equipment as well as in the structure of Company D. Ground ambulances and tents were eliminated. The aid station, as noted, was split into two sections. One section remained aboard the vessel at the rear anchorage; the other accompanied the combat units.

The two sections of the aid station were often separated for days. The section accompanying the combat units was split even further when two or three missions were conducted simultaneously in different areas. Since the physician attached to the company was almost always forward with the combat elements, the medical operations assistant, a Medical Service Corps officer, usually supervised the rear section at the base anchorage. This officer and the senior enlisted medical aidmen he supervised had considerably greater responsibility for the treatment and evacuation of patients than was customary. Casualties requiring more extensive care than could be provided in the rear section were evacuated by helicopter to a hospital. Helicopters as well as shuttle craft were used to supply the aid boats from the ship-based rear section. The rear section itself was supplied from shore.

4th Infantry Division

The 4th Infantry Division was deployed to Vietnam in July 1966. Each brigade moved by sea with all its supporting elements. Thus, the attached medical company was able to maintain a continuous record of the health of the command.

Although one brigade of the 4th Infantry Division was initially positioned in the coastal area of Phu Yen Province in III CTZ, the entire division was deployed to the Central Highlands by the end of 1966 to counter the steady buildup of North Vietnamese units in that region. During 1967, the division, and its predecessors in the Central Highlands, the 101st Airborne and the 25th Infantry Divisions, remained on the defensive. The brigades of these divisions were moved from one location to another in a series of spoiling operations as the need dictated, making it expedient at times to attach, detach, or exchange components of one division with those of another.

An example of this practice was the exchange between the 3d Brigade, 4th Infantry Division, and the 3d Brigade, 25th Infantry Division. The 3d Brigade, 25th Infantry Division, was operating in the Pleiku area when the 4th Infantry Division arrived in II CTZ. Thus it was assigned to the 4th Infantry Division along with its attached medical company. The 3d Brigade, 4th Infantry Division, and its attached medical company operated as a separate task force in the area of operations of the 25th Infantry Division. It was therefore inactivated and reactivated as the 3d Brigade, 25th Infantry Division. The exchange permitted direct operational control over these units. The medical companies exchanged became components of the medical battalions organic to their new divisions, the 4th and 25th Medical Battalions of the 4th and 25th Infantry Divisions, respectively.

Army-level medical support for the 1st Brigade, 4th Infantry Division, operating in the Tuy Hoa area, was provided by the 8th Field Hospital at Nha Trang. The 18th Surgical Hospital, supplemented by the 71st Evacuation Hospital in late 1967, serviced the main base camp at Pleiku.

United States forces in the Central Highlands went on the offensive in 1968 and 1969. Predicated on the mobility of the helicopter, landing zones and fire support bases were set up temporarily and operational sweeps were conducted from these sites. Since combat units were widely dispersed, it was necessary to subdivide the medical assets supporting them to insure the best coverage. The "light" clearing station was evolved for this purpose.

Under this concept, teams, each consisting of a physician and from seven to 10 medical enlisted men, deployed to the landing zones or fire support bases with the units they supported. These operations usually lasted from several days to several weeks. The forward area "light" clearing station worked in unison with the main components of the parent medical company at the semipermanent base camp in the rear where treatment facilities were housed in protected bunkers. The purpose of the "light" clearing station was to prepare the casualty for helicopter evacuation to the main section at the base camp. At this field station, casualties were quickly sorted out as to seriousness and type of wound to allow the worst cases to be evacuated first. An innovation in field medical service, the "light" clearing station allowed medical support to be provided concurrently at the base camp and in the field.

As combat activities diminished in 1970, the operations of the 4th Infantry Division were curtailed. In April 1970, the 3d Brigade, 4th Infantry Division, with its attached support elements, including Company D, 4th Medical Battalion, departed Vietnam for the continental United States. The other three companies of the 4th Medical Battalion remained in Vietnam to support the division base camp at Pleiku and the combat activities of the 1st and 2d Brigades of the division in the Central Highlands.

To support the mission of the 4th Infantry Division in the Cambodian incursion during May and June 1970, the 4th Medical Battalion positioned a clearing station at a fire support base close to the Cambodian border. Use of the six Dust-off helicopters assigned to support the clearing station was dictated by the nature of the operation. Two maintained an orbit over the landing zone, two remained on standby at the clearing station, and two were retained on call at the base camp. The majority of casualties from the Cambodian incursion received initial medical treatment at the 4th Medical Battalion's clearing station on the border.

23d (Americal) Infantry Division

Task Force OREGON, which later became the 23d (Americal) Infantry Division, was formed in April 1967. Operating from bases at Duc

Pho and Chu Lai, it moved into Quang Ngai and Quang Tin Provinces south of Da Nang along the coast. Its mission was to free Marine units operating in I CTZ South to reinforce the area southwest of Da Nang and near the Demilitarized Zone in I CTZ North where the enemy threat continued to grow in size and intensity throughout 1967.

The task force was composed of the 196th Light Infantry Brigade, the 3d Brigade, 25th Infantry Division (later the 3d Brigade, 4th Infantry Division), and the 1st Brigade, 101st Airborne Division. Formed as separate brigades, each had an attached medical company. Thus, the task force did not have a medical battalion. Medical planning and supply functions were provided by adding specialized administrative personnel to the staff of the task force surgeon, thus giving him the equivalent of a divisional medical battalion staff.

Task Force OREGON having accomplished its mission, the 23d (Americal) Infantry Division was formed in September 1967 for sustained combat operations in I CTZ. At that time, the 3d Brigade, 25th Infantry Division, and the 1st Brigade, 101st Airborne Division, were replaced by the 198th and 11th Light Infantry Brigades which had just arrived in Vietnam. These joined the 196th Light Infantry Brigade as organic components of the Americal Division. The 3d Brigade, 1st Cavalry Division (Airmobile), supported by Company A, 15th Medical Battalion (Airmobile), and the 3d Brigade, 4th Infantry Division, supported by Company D, 4th Medical Battalion, remained as attached units of the division. Initially, the 23d Medical Battalion, which was formed in December 1967 to support the Americal Division, operated with only a Headquarters and Company A since the other medical companies were organic to their brigades. When the Americal Division was reorganized under the ROAD (Reorganization Objective Army Divisions) concept in February 1969, three companies were added to the battalion and it was authorized a strength of 38 officers and 333 enlisted men.

Medical service in the Americal Division was a mixture of the old and the new. Casualties were evacuated from the forward area mainly by helicopter, but ground ambulances were used extensively for routine resupply, nonemergency patient evacuation, and to support MEDCAP (Medical Civic Action Program). Ground ambulances were also used extensively in the Chu Lai base area, which was more than 9 miles long, and by medical units stationed at brigade and battalion base areas along Route 1 in the Duc Pho and Chu Lai regions.

Since the size of the Americal Division's area of operations entailed fairly long air ambulance flights, medical companies were stationed at remote inland bases, such as Duc Pho. These companies retained sick and lightly wounded soldiers for early return to duty, and also provided emergency resuscitation of the severely wounded in preparation for the long helicopter flight to a hospital.

Battalion aid stations at the firebases were near the areas of extensive combat and could provide emergency medical treatment. Inclement weather often made it impossible to evacuate patients immediately, and the battalion surgeon was on hand to care for the seriously wounded. He was also available to advise the battalion commander on medical matters and, when necessary, could use the tactical communications net to assist his aidmen in the field.

Since there was no evacuation hospital in the Americal Division's area of operations—the nearest evacuation hospitals were located at Qui Nhon, more than 125 miles from Chu Lai—patients with predictable recovery rates were retained longer than normal at the medical clearing companies. Seriously wounded or critically ill patients were evacuated to the 2d Surgical Hospital or the 1st Marine Hospital Company at Chu Lai.

The companies of the 23d Medical Battalion were housed in semi-permanent installations. Throughout 1968 and 1969, patients were held for a period of 7 days at these clearing stations. At times, they were held longer, but this was the exception. Admissions to the clearing stations of the 23d Medical Battalion involving nonbattle injuries exceeded those resulting from hostile action; fever of undetermined origin was a primary cause for hospitalization.

The 23d Medical Battalion was also responsible for treating sick and wounded Vietnamese civilians. During the period from 1 January to 31 December 1969, the combined companies of the battalion treated 21,891 Vietnamese patients. While much of this treatment was outpatient care for the often neglected peasant in the villages and hamlets, a large percentage of more definitive medical, surgical, and rehabilitative treatment was done on the wards of the 23d Medical Battalion. Company B, 23d Medical Battalion, for example, maintained a civilian war casualty ward which accommodated 30 Vietnamese patients. The ward was constantly full and averaged about 110 patients a month. While constantly engaged in care of the sick and injured, the 23d Medical Battalion also conducted a vigorous program to train Vietnamese health workers so they could assume greater medical responsibilities in their own villages and hamlets.

Medical Support of Separate Infantry Brigades

Several brigade-sized units with organic or attached medical companies operated in Vietnam. These included the 11th, 196th, and 198th Light Infantry Brigades that later became the 23d (Americal) Infantry Division, with their organic medical companies still intact. Others were the 3d Brigade, 82d Airborne Division, the 3d Brigade, 5th Mechanized Division, the 199th Light Infantry Brigade, the 173d Airborne Brigade, and the 11th Armored Cavalry Regiment. The medical companies of these units operated independently of any higher headquarters in contrast to their divisional counterparts which were under the command of the division's medical battalion.

The medical companies of the 199th Light Infantry Brigade and the 173d Airborne Brigade were organic to their support battalions, the 6th and 173d Support Battalions, respectively. On the other hand, the 3d Brigade, 82d Airborne Division, and the 3d Brigade, 5th Mechanized Division, belonged to the division structures even though they operated as separate brigades. Therefore, their medical companies were attached and not organic. The 37th Medical Company, which supported the 11th Armored Cavalry Regiment, differed from the others in that it was neither an element of a support battalion nor a medical battalion. It had been specifically tailored for an armored cavalry regiment.

37th Medical Company

At the beginning of 1969, the function of the 37th Medical Company was to support the 11th Armored Cavalry Regiment operating in the Blackhorse area. Since all combat casualties from January through April 1969 were treated at the 7th Surgical Hospital, which was adjacent to the 37th Medical Company's clearing station, the company limited its activities to routine sick call and vigorous support of MEDCAP.

In May 1969, the 7th Surgical Hospital was inactivated. The 37th Medical Company inherited its superior facilities and reorganized its treatment capability considerably. The emergency room and ward were expanded, the dental clinic was enlarged, and an X-ray unit was installed. At the same time, a section was deployed to Quan Loi to support combat operations in the forward area.

When the 37th Medical Company was assigned the task of supporting the 3d Brigade, 1st Cavalry Division (Airmobile), which was also operating in the Blackhorse area, in May 1969, a mutual support program was established with Company C, 15th Medical Battalion (Airmobile), 1st Cavalry Division (Airmobile), with which the 37th Medical Company shared its facilities. During the summer months, the 37th Medical Company received an average of 2.7 casualties a day, who were evacuated to the rear clearing station by a medical evacuation helicopter from the 15th Medical Battalion (Airmobile). The superior facilites at this rear station, especially the X-ray unit that had been installed, permitted many less serious battle injuries to be treated entirely at the clearing station level. When the 199th Light Infantry Brigade replaced the 1st Cavalry Division (Airmobile), the 37th Medical Company, in co-operation with Company C, 7th Support Battalion, 199th Light Infantry Brigade, continued to provide routine sick call and casualty support in the area. Early in December 1969, the main body of the 37th Medical Company was deployed in Quan Loi to support the elements of the 11th Armored Cavalry Regiment. A small element was based at Bien Hoa to take advantage of access to the supply depot at Long Binh.

Task Force Shoemaker

Task Force SHOEMAKER, which participated in the Cambodian incursion, was composed of the 1st Brigade, 1st Cavalry Division (Airmobile); the 11th Armored Cavalry Regiment plus the 1st Squadron, 9th Cavalry Regiment; the 2d Battalion, 47th Mechanized Infantry Regiment; the 2d Battalion, 34th Armored Regiment; the 5th Battalion, 12th Infantry Regiment; and the 5th Battalion, 60th Infantry Regiment. The medical support of this operation illustrated the flexibility of the medical service in offensive sweeps by brigade-type units.

The task force received its medical support from elements of the 15th Medical Battalion (Airmobile) and the 37th Medical Company at the base camp at Quan Loi, near the center of the intended zone of operations. In addition two clearing stations in protected bunkers existed at this site. A forward command post of the 15th Medical Battalion (Airmobile) was added to Company C, 15th Medical Battalion, and the 37th Medical Company, the units operating the two clearing stations.

A special emergency medical team composed of a physician, two clinical technicians, three aidmen, and a radio operator was formed out of the Headquarters and Company A, 15th Medical Battalion (Airmobile). Available for duty anywhere in the task force's area of operations, it established a forward emergency treatment station at Katum where an aid station existed. Flown in with its equipment by helicopter, the team was functioning within an hour. A medical helicopter remained on station with the team.

In anticipation of many casualties, the bulk of the whole blood supply in Vietnam was moved forward for use by the 37th Medical Company and Company C, 15th Medical Battalion (Airmobile). The estimate of 500 to 800 casualties within the first 3 days of the operation failed to materialize, and the usable portion of the whole blood supply was returned to the 9th Medical Laboratory for redistribution.

The Air Ambulance Platoon, 15th Medical Battalion (Airmobile), moved up to Quan Loi for the operation. The platoon leader and his operations assistant were joined by the battalion commander, S-3, and an assistant of the 15th Medical Battalion (Airmobile) to co-ordinate the use of medical assets. Two helicopters were assigned to the 37th Medical Company in direct support of the 11th Armored Cavalry Regiment while three others operated out of Quan Loi with Company C, 15th Medical Battalion (Airmobile). Other medical evacuation helicopters were stationed at landing zones and fire support bases. A Dust-off helicopter remained on standby at Quan Loi to evacuate casualties from the clearing station to a hospital.

After 4 days, the task force was dissolved and the 1st Cavalry Division (Airmobile) took over the operational control of all the former components of the task force. Operations shifted eastward inside of Cambodia north of Bu Dop. A second emergency medical team from Headquarters and Company A, 15th Medical Battalion (Airmobile), was emplaced at Bu Dop.

To summarize the operation, the 15th Medical Battalion (Airmobile) moved a "jump" command post forward to Quan Loi, which consisted of the battalion commander, S–3, an assistant, and the air ambulance platoon leader and his operations officer. Two emergency medical teams were established, one at Katum and one at Bu Dop. Each team treated about 30 emergency cases. The air ambulances of the 15th Medical Battalion (Airmobile) were positioned at a variety of places within the area of operations to insure adequate evacuation capability. The 45th Medical Company (Air Ambulance) provided one helicopter on standby at Quan Loi for the backhaul missions in addition to a liaison officer in the forward area with the medical battalion. This arrangement proved to be one of the key factors in providing the best possible medical care to the combat troops involved in the Cambodian operation.

Trial Reorganization

By mid-summer of 1967, it was apparent that the impact of the helicopter on the doctrine and organization of field medical service was not transitory. The almost exclusive reliance upon the helicopter ambulance had virtually eliminated the battalion aid station, and often the division clearing station, from the chain of evacuation when a surgical, evacuation, or field hospital was within the same flying time or distance.

Many medical officers with combat experience in Vietnam agreed that the reliance upon the helicopter was not a condition that was limited to the peculiarities of the Vietnam conflict. Enough experience in a variety of operations over the previous 2 years had been accumulated to support the belief that the time had come to conduct the appropriate tests so that modifications could be instituted. A hundred physicians were interviewed in the field, often under combat conditions, as to their recommendations. Their reports were analyzed along with the critiques that had been solicited over the previous 2 years.

It was apparent that realignment of personnel and organization was needed to allow for a more efficient application of medical assets. The consensus was that there were too many physicians in the division and brigade medical organization to make full use of their talents. Plans for a new alignment were developed and tested by the 1st Infantry Division from October 1967 into March of the following year. It was estimated, on the basis of the test, that the number of physicians in the division could be reduced from 34 to approximately 12 without impairing the quality of medical care available to the troops.

During the test period, the brigade surgeon, artillery battalion surgeon, and engineer battalion surgeon positions were eliminated. The artillery and engineer battalions retained their medical sections as did the aviation battalion and cavalry squadron. The medical battalion was moved from the support command to division control and the infantry battalion medical platoons were placed under its direct command. Thus the medical battalion commander controlled all medical resources.

As a result of the test, all the brigade, artillery, and engineer surgeon positions were eliminated from the division medical organization. One-half of the wheeled ambulances and their crews were eliminated from the medical battalion while the medical platoons of the infantry battalions were reassigned to it. Operational control of the entire division medical service was delegated to the division surgeon.

Exact utilization of medical officers varied with each division and brigade, but by the end of 1970, all were operating under the general concept that physicians should not be assigned to combat and combat support units.

CHAPTER VII

Aviation Medicine

Approximately two-thirds of the Army aviation resources supporting operations in Vietnam were assigned to the units of the 1st Aviation Brigade. The remaining aircraft and men were assigned to those units organic to the divisions; relatively few were assigned to artillery, engineer, aircraft maintenance, signal, or other support units. Although the strength of the 1st Aviation Brigade was not much greater than 25,000 men, its approximately 50 flight surgeons provided primary medical care on an area basis to more than 35,000 troops. In some areas, the dispensaries of the 1st Aviation Brigade were the only source of outpatient care. The medical units of the brigade established liaison and close working relationships with their nearest supporting hospitals, referring patients for consultations, inpatient care, and specialized treatment.

The flight surgeon is a physician who has received formal training in the specialized field of aviation medicine. His mission includes the prevention and treatment of disease, injury, and mental or emotional deterioration among aviation flight, ground crew, and maintenance personnel. He monitors the programs of flyers and is expected to participate in frequent flights. He is confronted by the problems of traumatic injury; of acute and chronic disease, ranging from the common upper respiratory infections to the most uncommon of tropical diseases; of psychiatric disorders, which run the gamut from occupational fatigue through the minor disorders of personality to overt psychoses; and of personal hygiene and environmental sanitation, including dietetics, venereal disease, insect control, and a multitude of bizarre and homely worrisome matters. The flight surgeon treats physical and mental conditions that might endanger pilots or passengers. Whether in the examination room or upon the flight line, he must be able readily to detect incipient major and minor disorders of personality in men who, in their zeal to fly, frequently try to conceal the disorders. He administers and prescribes medications and treatment, and he reviews and studies the case history and the progress of the patient. He also acts as consultant in his specialty to other medical services and provides aeromedical staff advice. In addition, the flight surgeon serves as medical member of aircraft crash investigation teams and, when possible, contributes to aeromedical research and development.

The number of flight surgeons authorized in Vietnam reached a maximum of 86 in August 1968; by November, 98 were actually assigned there. This maximum contrasted with shortages during such periods as August 1967, when these assignments fell to 40 percent below the authorized strength.

The flight surgeon, assigned to a unit of an aviation brigade, was supported by a medical detachment team which provided dispensary service. These teams were assigned generally on a basis of one detachment per two aviation companies. The unit flight dispensary was usually located next to the airfield, often in a unit billeting area, and the flight surgeon and his staff usually lived with the troops that they served. This arrangement, allowing for optimum rapport and medical services, was especially advantageous when the airfields were under attack, and it proved vital during the 1968 Tet Offensive, when many airfields were isolated.

Flyer Fatigue

The aeromedical problems that faced Army aviation units in Vietnam provided a challenge to their supporting flight surgeons. No problem, however, was more common yet more elusive than that of flyer fatigue. It became more pronounced after 1965 when the buildup of U.S. forces gained momentum and remained a significant limiting factor in the conduct of airmobile operations. By the end of 1966, aviators were flying 100 to 150 hours or more per month, and the need to know how much an aviator could fly before he was so fatigued that he was no longer effective or safe was evident.

Army aviators were assailed by a multitude of stresses, each to some extent capable of endangering their missions. The stress from hostile fire was aggravated by such factors as heat, dehydration, noise, vibration, blowing dust, hazardous weather, exhaust from engines and weapons, and labyrinthine stimulation. Additional stress was caused by psychic elements, such as fear, insufficient sleep, family separation, and frustration. These stresses, acting on the aviator day after day, combined with the physical exertion of long hours of piloting an aircraft, caused fatigue.

The ever-increasing requirements during the years 1967–68 for aviation support caused the accrual of extremely high aviator flying times in all units. Night operations, with their extra demand upon the critical judgment of the aviator, increased. The shortage of crews often forced an individual to undertake both day and night missions without adequate rest.

In response to expressed concern of the unit commanders and of aviation safety officers, flight surgeons at all levels of aeromedical support studied every aspect of the fatigue problem. Because fatigue was the result of many variables, it defied easy definition and precise measurement.

Emphasis, therefore, was placed on prevention—eliminating or reducing those factors in the aviator's environment that caused stress.

General Neel, Surgeon, USARV, noted in the Command Health Report for August 1968 that approximately 70 percent of aircraft accidents were found to be the result of pilot error and that pilot fatigue had been implicated as a contributing factor in a large proportion of accidents. He indicated that the only way to cope with pilot fatigue was prevention by reducing the aviator's flying hours. His recommendation was "that immediate action be taken to provide additional aviators to USARV insuring at least 100 percent authorized aviator strength to reduce the degree to which pilot fatigue is contributing to the loss of lives and expensive aircraft." This was never done.

The unit flight surgeon's close scrutiny of charts that showed each pilot's flying hours for the previous 30 days, followed by close co-operation among the unit commander, platoon leaders, operations officer, noncommissioned officers, and flight surgeon, proved an invaluable system for collecting data on which the flight surgeon based his final recommendation to the commander. By the end of 1968, this system was utilized by most of the aviation units.

Some flight surgeons, notably Captain Philip Snodgrass, MC, of the 269th Aviation Battalion at Cu Chi, believed that the relationship of days flown to days off and, particularly, the provision of a scheduled "on-off" work cycle were more important than the total number of hours flown. Captain Snodgrass's staff study of a "goal-directed" flying-hour schedule indicated that a series of 5 or 6 days flown, followed by a scheduled day free from flying and from other duties, resulted in a unit that evidenced less fatigue and could fly even greater numbers of hours. This idea was adopted by many units and proved workable and effective.

Fatigue in the enlisted crew members was a less obvious, though very real, threat. These individuals, who accompanied the aircraft on all its missions, returned to their base camps only to work many additional hours in providing required maintenance and preparing for the following day's missions. With the added requirement of aiding in perimeter defense and in the multitudinous other details of combat aviation, they performed under great stress. Efforts by the unit flight surgeons in their behalf centered upon improving their living conditions, eliminating some extra duties, and increasing their numbers.

By 1970, fatigue as an entity was still no better defined nor more capable of measurement than before. Moreover, the attempt at limiting aviator flying hours by regulation had been proved ineffective in the combat environment, and the requirement for continued study of the problem was evidently needed.

Care of the Flyer Program

Flight Physicals

The problem of performing periodic physical examinations on flying personnel began with the first Army aviation unit in Vietnam. Equipment and facilities were not available for an adequate examination. This handicap was partially overcome by Department of the Army waiver of the requirement for routine periodic examinations for rated aviators in Vietnam; however, despite the waiver, many still requested them. Periodic examinations for crew chiefs, flight surgeons, and aerial observers were also waived; required initial examinations were performed as well as available equipment allowed. Modifications of organization and the addition of equipment helped eliminate these difficulties. Aerial door gunners were not given a complete examination. After reviewing their medical records, the flight surgeon gave them a general examination which included visual tests and their "Adaptability Rating for Military Aeronautics." A statement of medical qualification was then issued by the flight surgeon.

Waiver authority was retained by USARV headquarters for medical standards for pilots, crew chiefs, flight surgeons, and aerial observers. Headquarters policy on standards for pilots was strict. Policy on standards for others who were expected to participate in aerial flights was considerably more lenient; conditions were waived if they were not dangerous to the individual's health and would not interfere with mission completion.

Significant Medical Conditions

The incidence of infectious disease among aviation personnel in Vietnam generally paralleled that of other troops in the area. Many diseases, however, were more serious for flying personnel because of possible time lost from primary duties. Basic preventive medicine, therefore, was of prime importance to the unit flight surgeon.

Diarrhea and upper respiratory infections were particularly costly in terms of aviator availability. Aviation companies normally operated a single mess and, on some occasions, were rendered ineffective for short periods because of epidemic gastroenteritis. Food and ice procured from local handlers were frequent sources of these outbreaks despite constant screening and surveillance by the flight surgeon. Venereal diseases, notably gonorrhea, were of particularly high incidence.

Breakdowns in basic field medicine practices and water supply control occurred. Individual soldiers were occasionally charged with the treatment of water without adequate knowledge of the techniques involved. Failure to maintain adequate chlorine residual and even the accidental use of nonpotable supplies presented problems. In April 1968, in the 1st Cavalry Division (Airmobile), thousands of cases of gastroenteritis severe enough to cause loss from duty occurred almost simultaneously, and many more men were symptomatic without loss of duty. Investigation implicated contaminated water. The 164th Aviation Group, located in the Delta region with headquarters at Can Tho, had outbreaks of hepatitis during the summers of 1967, 1968, and 1969. Mass immunization with gamma globulin was required to abort these episodes, some of which apparently originated from using nonpotable ice and frequenting Vietnamese food establishments.

Aircrews frequently encountered skin disorders, often miliarial or fungal in etiology. The long hours of flying while dressed in protective equipment and the intense dust clouds raised by helicopter operations contributed to the adverse dermatological environment. External otitis sometimes caused restriction of flying duties.

Malaria was significant only sporadically. Basic mosquito control measures were effective in secure base areas, and it was there that aircrews usually spent their evenings. The continuous presence of the aviation unit flight surgeon with constant emphasis on preventive medicine techniques and health education for the aviator undoubtedly contributed to the low incidence.

Medication and Therapy

Traditional aeromedical philosophy on the use of drugs by flying personnel is conservative. AR 40-501 and AR 40-8 specifically limit their use. The flight surgeon's duty was to promote a state of individual fitness that allowed the flyer to meet the myriad stresses of combat flying. Ideally, the use of systemic therapeutic agents should have been prohibited in Vietnam, as they are elsewhere, but realistically, the unit commander needed the maximum number of personnel to carry out his mission. It was the duty of the flight surgeons to evaluate the risk of using therapeutic and prophylactic agents against the impact of losing personnel to flying duties while undergoing treatment. On this basis, the flight surgeon frequently administered certain drugs without restricting the aviator from flying, and other drugs after careful evaluation of the pilot's condition and his particular response to the drug. When the acute medical condition of an aircrewman did not prohibit flying status, he was often allowed to fly after a period of drug use to determine his susceptibility to side effects. Antibiotics and decongestants were used but antihistaminics, sedatives, and tranquilizers were prohibited.

Aviation personnel had to take the weekly malaria chemoprophylactic tablet; those who exhibited significant side effects were evaluated by the unit flight surgeon and placed on chloroquine tablets if the reaction was due to the primaquine component. Many aviation units required their men to take the chloroquine-primaquine tablet on Monday night rather than on Monday morning because of the diarrhea that sometimes occurred shortly after ingestion. The incidence of glucose-6-phosphate dehydrogenase deficiency was low.

Dapsone, when introduced in Vietnam, was used only where recommended by the appropriate medical authority; a very low incidence of methemoglobinemia was evaluated in the 7/17th Air Cavalry Squadron by the unit flight surgeon and the WRAIR team in Saigon. The incidence of fungus infections prompted therapy with griseofulvin in selected aviators, who continued to fly during long-term treatment. Throughout the years of Army aviation operations in Vietnam, the practical approach to the question of therapeutic agents turned out to be effective.

Safety

Accidental injury was a source of significant personnel loss. Aircraft accidents, until the spring of 1968, caused more aircrew injury and death than did enemy action. Less spectacular but also significant were those casualties caused by weapons accidents, vehicle mishaps, and sports. Relatively simple injuries removed the patients from flying duties for the duration of treatment.

All flight surgeons participated in the flight safety program at all levels of command. In addition to their constant fatigue monitoring and their vigilant protection of the mental, emotional, and physical health of all aircrews, they served as advisers in evaluating and proposing protective armor for both aircraft and aircrew.

Aircrew Wound Experience

The vulnerability of the helicopter when used as a tactical aircraft is extremely serious. The ways in which the vulnerability of the crew may be reduced is a significant matter. During 1965 and 1966, studies were made on the effectiveness of armor for both men and equipment. Although helicopter crashes frequently were caused by enemy fire, evidence existed that few were the result of injury to the pilot. By the end of 1965, crashes had caused 101 fatal and 79 nonfatal injuries, and "missiles and shells" had caused 43 fatal and 673 nonfatal wounds. Effectiveness of seat armor was implicit in the notation "most fatalities due to wounds of head, throat, and upper torso."

Medical input requested by the 1966 Army Materiel Command study group for a study in Vietnam was provided by representatives of

USAMRDC (U.S. Army Medical Research and Development Command).

In April 1966, Captain James W. Ralph, MC, produced a staff study on aviation casualty reporting for the Army Concept Team in Vietnam in an attempt to determine whether or not the data being compiled was being analyzed and could be applied to studies of protective equipment. With the collaboration of Major (later Colonel) James E. Hertzog, MC, Surgeon, 1st Aviation Brigade, and Aviation Medicine Consultant, USARV, a form was developed for reporting wounds.

In June 1966, USARV Regulation 40-42, "Wound Evaluation and Analysis," was published, requiring that specific data be reported on all crewmembers wounded in Vietnam, and placing the responsibility for implementation upon the unit flight surgeon. By early 1967, only a small percent of wound incidence had been reported because of communication and transportation difficulties. The number and locations of the medical facilities hindered the flight surgeons' interviewing and recording the pertinent data on every wounded aircrewman. Late in the year, the regulation was amended to provide for reporting by the commander of the medical facility receiving an injured aircrewman; the amendment resulted only in total failure of the reporting system. Although the amount of wound data reported by flight surgeons in 1966 was meager, the available information showed that both personnel armor and aircraft armor were of great protective value.

Life Support Equipment

At the onset of Army aviation operations in Vietnam, crewmembers flew their support missions in H-21 aircraft, dressed in fatigues or U.S. Air Force issue coveralls, leather gloves, and 1959 model APH-5 flight helmets. With the exception of occasional flak jackets of Korean War vintage, any additional protection was provided by makeshift means. The aircraft were not armored and were relatively vulnerable to enemy fire. In general, survival kits were also makeshift. The need for measures to increase the survivability of aircrewmembers was evident.

In 1962, the Army Materiel Command initiated a long-term research and development project to reduce the vulnerability of Army aircraft and aircrew. The results of this project and the related efforts of other commands, such as USAMRDC, provided much of the equipment lacking in those early years. Flight surgeons in the field provided impetus to this development effort.

While crash-injury fatalities in aircraft hit by ground fire were three times those caused by bullet wounds, the need for protection from small arms fire was recognized through work done by the U.S. Army Ballistic Research Laboratories. By 1965, the H-21 helicopters had been phased out of Vietnam, and all UH–1 aircraft were equipped with armored seats for the pilot and copilot. Unfortunately, the great need for an armored seat for the gunner and crew chief on UH–1 aircraft was never met in the field, although development was undertaken.

Body armor of bullet-protective plates in a canvas carrier was introduced in 1965 for protection of the torso. It was widely accepted by aircrews. The pilot and copilot of the aircraft utilized the chest protection only, since they were otherwise protected by the armored seat. Body armor containing both front and back protective plates was worn by other crewmen of the aircraft. There are many documented cases of individuals sustaining direct hits on these protective plates without injury other than bruises.

In January 1966, the Department of the Army approved a project for the development of flight clothing which would provide fire protection, be compatible with cockpit design, and resemble the uniform worn by the foot soldier. Deliveries to Vietnam of a two-piece Nomex uniform began early in 1968, and by year's end adequate quantities were on hand to meet all requirements. In 1969, the fire-resistant flight uniform, having been well received by aircrews, was made Standard A for the Army.

Individually carried survival kits were considered necessary by most flight surgeons and aircrewmen in Vietnam early in the war. A variety of survival kits were developed and made available in quantity. However, as experience accumulated in Vietnam, it was noted that survival kits were seldom utilized by the survivors of downed aircraft. Few persons were rescued if downed in hostile territory more than a few hours. The consensus of flight surgeons and other aeromedical personnel was that items of signal equipment were most valuable. The survival radio, if working, appeared to be the most important item in the location and rescue of downed aircrewmen. Recognition of this fact led to emphasis upon the continuing development of more reliable survival radio sets.

Before 1961, flight surgeons had cited the need for better head protection, including fragmentation protection. Early in 1967, after more than 6 years of development, the AFH–1 helmet, which met specifications, was delivered to aviation units but proved to be too small for many of the aircrewmen. Major (later Lieutenant Colonel) Anthony A. Bezreh, MC, who, as aviation medicine consultant and 1st Aviation Brigade surgeon, had provided primary impetus to the improvement of items of safety equipment, reported the results of a survey done on this helmet. Later attempts at modifying it were largely unsuccessful, and until 1969, aircrews were wearing a mixture of APH–5 and AFH–1 helmets.

In 1969, a new flight helmet, the SPH–4, incorporating markedly improved retention and noise attenuation qualities, was procured for use in Vietnam and received immediate acceptance in the field. It proved effective in the prevention of injuries and became Standard A early in 1970.

CHAPTER VIII

Preventive Medicine

The Preventive Medicine Division, Office of the Surgeon, USARV, was organized late in 1965 to advise the command on the incidence, prevalence, and epidemiological aspects of diseases which were likely to occur among U.S. Army combat soldiers and, therefore, to be hazardous to military operations in Vietnam.

The 20th Preventive Medicine Unit (Field), formerly the 20th Preventive Medicine Laboratory, was the first preventive medicine unit deployed to Vietnam. Originally this unit and later four preventive medicine detachments functioned independently, but late in 1967, higher echelon technical support was required and the four detachments were assigned to the 20th Preventive Medicine Unit which then assumed responsibility for the countrywide U.S. Army preventive medicine program. When the 172d Preventive Medicine Unit (Field) became operational on 29 July 1968, the responsibility for preventive medicine support in Vietnam was divided between the two units. Both units were assigned to the 44th Medical Brigade, and each was augmented by two detachments, one control team and one survey team. Thus, countrywide deployment followed, from Quang Tri in the north to Can Tho in the south.

Communicable Diseases

Malaria

Steady progress in the reduction of malaria in Vietnam had been possible through vigorous command emphasis, improved preventive regimens, and increased control measures. A major change in the chloroquine-primaquine chemoprophylaxis program was instituted with Change 1 to USARV Regulation 40–4. This change stipulated that units in high-risk areas were to take daily dapsone tablets in addition to weekly chloroquine-primaquine tablets as chemoprophylaxis against *Plasmodium falciparum*, the malarial parasite responsible for nearly 98 percent of infections occurring among troops. The command surgeon notified field commanders to enforce this change when manpower losses due to infections with *P. falciparum* were greater than 20 cases per 1,000 per annum per major unit.

The Wilson-Edeson test, adopted by the 172d Preventive Medicine Unit, to measure the amount of chloroquine in urine, was rapid and convenient for field use. This test helped field commanders evaluate objectively each unit's malaria chemoprophylaxis program and resulted in a dramatic drop in the malaria rate in the units tested. Since slightly more than 80 percent of all cases of malaria occurred in combat units, it was the responsibility of field commanders to provide consistent and continuous command emphasis on preventive measures. In addition to chloroquine-primaquine and dapsone chemoprophylaxis, personal protective measures to control malaria were stressed. Skin repellents, aerosol insecticide dispensers, bednets, and headnets were in general use by field units. Combat units in remote forward areas received repellents and aerosol dispensers routinely.

For personnel departing Vietnam, commanders were urged to insure that the malaria chemoprophylaxis records of all returnees were reviewed as soon as possible after arrival at their new duty station to make certain that each returnee had signed a "malaria debriefing" statement. This procedure was recommended to prevent manpower loss and to limit the spread of malaria from infected soldiers to susceptible persons in the United States and other areas. Those individuals who had not completed the 8-week chloroquine-primaquine course and the 28-day dapsone course were to be given sufficient tablets to complete the malaria chemoprophylaxis course they were on in Vietnam.

Infectious Hepatitis

Beginning in 1966, all troops in Vietnam were inoculated with gamma globulin during their first and fifth months of assignment to control infectious hepatitis. Later, as the troop strength increased, a system of selective priorities was set up for the use of this serum, based upon the premise of the greatest need. Most cases of infectious hepatitis were caused by eating or drinking contaminated food or water. The disease was of special concern when those infected were cooks or food handlers. Continuous efforts were made to inform all troops of the dangers inherent in consuming food purchased on the economy, where contact with the virus was unavoidable.

Diarrheal Diseases

The most common disease among U.S. soldiers in Vietnam was diarrhea. The rate for this disease showed seasonal variations with peaks each year during May and June, but the greater number of cases were sporadic and were usually caused by a breakdown in unit mess sanitation or by eating locally procured vegetables contaminated with *Shigella* and *Salmonella*. No specific etiological agent was identified for most of the diarrheal cases admitted for treatment. Shigellosis accounted for most cases for which an agent could be identified.

Measures were continued to improve mess and water sanitation and waste disposal practices, and to educate the soldiers in basic field and food sanitation. The use of disposable paper plates and plastic eating utensils eradicated a potential source of diarrheal disease—inadequately cleaned mess gear.

Skin Disease

Skin disease caused by prolonged exposure to wetness followed by secondary invasion of the injured tissue by fungal or bacterial agents was a problem among U.S. Army ground troops fighting in inundated areas during the monsoon season. The Office of the Surgeon, USARV, recommended that all combat units be provided with zipper boots, inserts, and nylon socks. The most useful preventive measures were limiting participation in combat operations in wet areas to 48 hours, intensive foot care during the "drying out" period which followed, frequent changes of boots and socks, and prophylactic use of griseofulvin.

Fever of Undetermined Origin

Fever of undetermined origin was a major cause of morbidity in Vietnam. Elaborate studies were initiated before 1966 in an attempt to identify the etiological agent or agents involved. By 1968, through laboratory efforts, 40 percent of the admissions were identified as caused by arboviruses or other arthropodborne agents. The preventive measures used were insect sprays and bednets.

Rabies

As the U.S. Army troop buildup in Vietnam increased, there was a concomitant rise in the number of animal bite cases treated in USARV medical facilities. The major difficulties were the sheer number of pets acquired by Americans, the large number of small units and detachments scattered among the Vietnamese communities, and the lack of a meaningful civilian rabies control program. There were no cases of rabies among USARV personnel during 1965–70, although several thousand soldiers received the antirabies vaccine prophylaxis when the biting animal was not apprehended.

To control rabies in pets, the preventive medicine rabies control program required that each unit commander determine the number of animals to be allowed in his area, that all animals be registered, and that each animal be vaccinated against rabies and restrained within the unit area. Little restraint of pets was ever noted in Vietnam.

Other Communicable Diseases

Other communicable diseases of special concern occurred in Vietnam and could have become a threat with the increase of troop strength and acceleration of combat operations without an effective preventive medicine program.

The admission rates for common respiratory disease and influenza remained relatively moderate from 1965 to 1970. Although an outbreak of influenza in Hong Kong in July 1968 was caused by a strain of influenza virus sufficiently different to warrant concern over a probable pandemic, only a few cases appeared in military units in Vietnam. The monovalent vaccine became available in limited amounts in January and February 1969.

Melioidosis, a glanders-like disease observed in rodents and occasionally in man, was rarely encountered by the Army before deployment of troops to Vietnam. *Pseudomonas pseudomallei*, the causative agent of melioidosis, was cultured from samples of oil, market fruits and vegetables, well water, and surface water. These may have been the source of infection since man-to-man transmission was not observed. Recognition and early treatment were the prime factors in reducing the melioidosis mortality rate in 1968.

Dengue fever was reported in small numbers during 1966, and scrub typhus cases in even fewer numbers. Immunization against typhus, routine since late 1962, was temporarily discontinued on 25 February 1969, because available vaccines were not potent enough to protect individuals against louseborne typhus fever.

Although both cholera and plague were prevalent during 1966 among the civil population of Vietnam, no cases of cholera occurred among U.S. troops from 1965 to 1970. As of 19 April 1968, five confirmed cases of plague and one unconfirmed case had occurred among U.S. Army personnel.

Environmental Sanitation

Field Sanitation Training

Instructors in preventive medicine units and detachments continuously stressed basic hygiene and sanitation, malaria chemoprophylaxis, insect and pest control, waste disposal, and unit and individual protective measures against arthropodborne and waterborne diseases as well as other health hazards that caused discomfort to troops or damage to materiel.

Water Supply Surveillance

Major emphasis was placed on medical surveillance of field water points and cantonment water supply systems. Preventive medicine units provided first-echelon surveillance of water supplies for organizations without assigned medical personnel, and second-echelon surveillance of water supplies for all others. The USARV requirement for free available chlorine in water was strictly enforced: 5.0 parts per million after 30 minutes contact at field water points and 2.0 parts per million at field consumption points.

Preventive medicine units also provided medical surveillance of iceplants, including residual chlorine and bacteriological testing of the quality of water. Ice consumed or used for chilling foods and beverages was supplied by iceplants operated by the Army or by Army-approved local civilian firms.

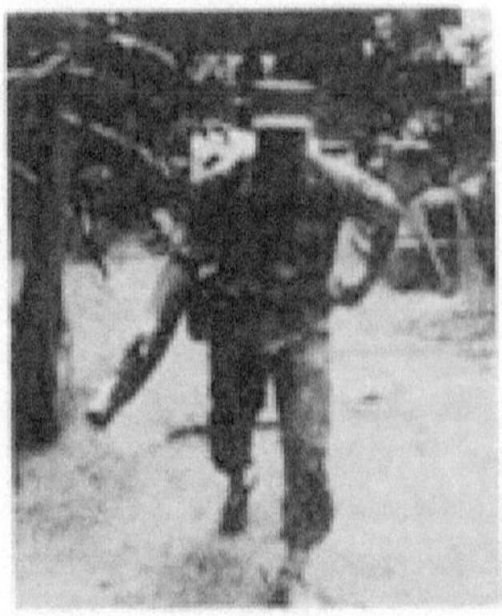

PREVENTIVE MEDICINE UNIT TEAM MEMBER USING THE MITEY MITE BACKPACK SPRAYER-DUSTER

Waste Disposal Practice

Monitoring waste disposal practices was another important preventive medicine activity; no major breakdowns in the waste disposal systems were related to disease outbreaks. In general, field units used urine soakage pits, with or without "urineoils," and "burn-out" latrines for the disposal of human excreta. For liquid wastes, oxidation ponds and sewage lagoons were used as well as septic tanks with soil absorption beds. Refuse—garbage, trash, kitchen wastes—was disposed of in sanitary fills. Infectious wastes from hospitals and other medical facilities were disposed of in high-temperature incinerators or by special packaging and burial.

Food Service Sanitation

Messkit sanitation procedures were almost totally unnecessary in Vietnam. Troops provided with rations used plastic trays, paper plates, or, in rare cases, chinaware. The individual combat meal (C-ration) was usually eaten with the utensils provided with the ration. The use of food service disinfectants, an item of special interest for USARV annual general inspections, was emphasized.

Pest Control Measures

Pest control in USARV was an integrated program involving the co-ordinated efforts of unit field sanitation teams, contract engineer entomology services, and preventive medicine units and detachments. Unit self-help sparked by trained field sanitation teams was the backbone of the program. In addition to pest control, preventive medicine personnel provided first- and second-echelon support to unit programs and insured that field sanitation teams were trained. Contract engineer entomology services were provided at major installations and base camps throughout Vietnam by Pacific Architects and Engineers and by the Philco Ford Company. Preventive medicine units conducted ground fogging and mist operations in remote areas where contract entomology services were lacking. Close liaison and co-operation were encouraged by medical entomologists with engineer entomologists to insure rapid exchange of information. The engineer program was unique in that it was the first time in recent history that the mission of pest control had been given on a broad scale to a civilian contractor in a combat zone.

Quarantine and Inspection Procedures

Early in the 1960's, the Armed Forces Pest Control Board was designated the co-ordinating agency for development of appropriate insect and rodent control programs for the Armed Forces. The Armed Forces had become increasingly aware of the real threat of accidental importation into the United States from Vietnam of pests and diseases of agricultural and medical concern. The inherent problems of inspecting vast quantities of cargo at U.S. ports of entry demanded the establishment of a preshipment quarantine inspection program for military cargo. Quarantine inspection of vessels, aircraft, and retrograde cargo in Vietnam was part of a co-operative preventive medicine program between the Department of Defense, the USPHS (U.S. Public Health Service), and the USDA (U.S. Department of Agriculture), during 1969. More than 350 medical personnel of the Army, Navy, and Air Force were trained and certified as USPHS and USDA quarantine inspectors. A 24-hour daily inspection service was maintained at major maritime and aerial ports operated by the Armed Forces for incoming and outgoing cargo. In addition, by special arrangement, cargo shipments were inspected and certified at auxiliary ports located throughout Vietnam.

Professional Conferences

Three USARV preventive medicine conferences were held during a 12-month period in 1968 and 1969. These 1-day conferences were conducted as working seminars and included formal presentations and informal study groups. About 75 individuals attended each conference. Besides participants from all USARV commands, there were preventive medicine representatives of the Surgeon, USMACV; AID; and ARVN. The seminars and panel discussions covered all phases of preventive medicine and provided the means for exchange of information and the opportunity to profit from the experience of personnel in different areas of Vietnam.

CHAPTER IX

The Military Blood Program

Time is crucial in the collection, delivery, and distribution of whole blood for large numbers of traumatic casualties. From 1965 forward, the stimulus behind the plans for a whole blood distribution program to support U.S. forces in the war in Vietnam was the need for speed. Blood is perishable, and its useful life is short. From donor to patient, liquified whole blood has a life expectancy of 21 days. Still, the most desirable blood for transfusion is the freshest blood available of the group and type specific for the recipient, completely and accurately processed and cross matched—a combination of perfections difficult to achieve in war.

Evolution of the System

The dominant conviction of the early blood program planners in USARPAC and USARV was that whole blood requires professional surveillance in handling from the moment it is drawn from the donor until the moment it is administered to the patient. Contaminated blood can be lethal.

By 1965 and the buildup of forces in Vietnam, the time had come to move with haste. Fortunately for the planners, requirements for whole blood increased slowly in 1965 and not with the same explosive force experienced at the beginning of the Korean War. Another asset was the substantial number of directives and guides already written and the existence of the Military Blood Program Agency.

Colonel Neel, Surgeon, USMACV, Major (later Colonel) Frank W. Kiel, MC, Commanding Officer, 406th Mobile Medical Laboratory, Vietnam, and Colonel Joseph F. Metzger, MC, Commanding Officer, 406th Medical Laboratory, Japan, in late 1965, were guided by three major principles based on experience gained thus far in the collection, processing, handling, and distribution of blood for troops in Vietnam. These medical officers, however, could not envision that requirements for whole blood would climb slowly but steadily from less than 100 units per month in 1965 to 8,000 units by February 1966, skyrocket to more than 30,000 units per month by 1968, peak at 38,000 units in February 1969, and fall rapidly to less than 15,000 units by mid-1970. (*Chart 12*)

CHART 12—UNITS OF BLOOD AVAILABLE IN SOUTH VIETNAM, BY MONTH, JANUARY 1965–DECEMBER 1970 [1]

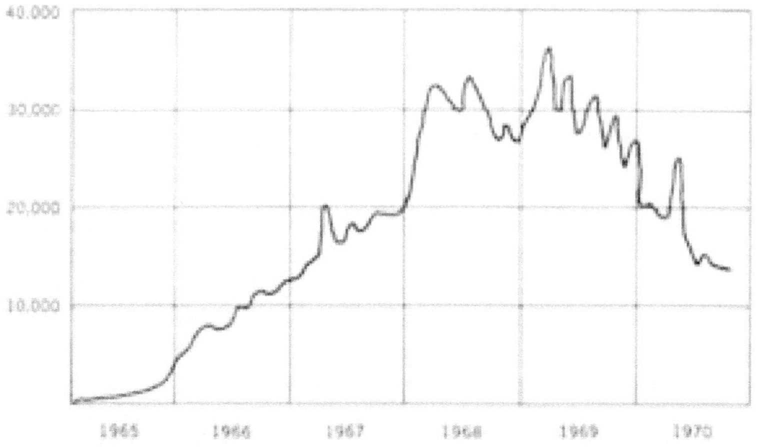

[1] Includes shipments from the continental United States, the Pacific Command, and blood collected in South Vietnam.

Source: Report, U.S. Military Whole Blood Program in Support of Combat Operations, South Vietnam, 1965–1970, prepared for the Deputy Surgeon General, February 1971.

The first guiding principle was that a source of whole blood outside Vietnam and the Pacific Command was essential. Donor resources in the Pacific could not meet the demands for whole blood during the buildup. Second was the establishment of a central depot in Saigon where all whole blood shipped from Japan could be received, transshipped, and distributed for use in the field. Third was the need for a system of forward mobile blood storage subdepots operated by the Army and colocated with hospitals and medical units in the Army, Navy, and Air Force along the South Vietnam coast.

A single American hospital in Vietnam, the 8th Field Hospital, administered all whole blood transfusions until the spring of 1965. Every 10 days, 10 units of universal donor low titer group O blood were shipped to the hospital from Japan to meet the small demand for transfusions. Seldom did the demand for blood exceed the supply, and even during the surprise attacks by the Vietcong at Qui Nhon and Pleiku, in February 1965, the 406th Mobile Medical Laboratory bled local donors to supply the needed 123 units of whole blood. After the 3d Field Hospital arrived in Saigon in May 1965, it became the central blood depot in Vietnam, and the 406th Mobile Medical Laboratory, a satellite of the 406th Medical Laboratory in Japan, was charged with distributing whole blood to all U.S. forces in Vietnam.

In the meantime, with the expanding need for blood, reorganization of the whole blood program for PACOM (Pacific Command) was underway. Colonel Metzger was also designated Blood Program Officer, PACOM, with direct responsibility to CINCUSARPAC (Commander in Chief, U.S. Army, Pacific) for the co-ordination and integration of plans, policies, and procedures to insure blood for all areas in USARPAC, including USARV.

The embryonic whole blood distribution system in Vietnam continued to expand and by 1967 was serving all Free World forces in Vietnam, excluding the RVN Army which met its own blood needs. The responsibility for supervising and operating the central blood bank in Vietnam came under the technical direction of Colonel Hinton J. Baker, MC, Commanding Officer, 9th Medical Laboratory, 3d Field Hospital, Saigon. The USARV Central Blood Bank operated under the parent laboratory's 9th Medical Laboratory Detachment and was supported by personnel from the 3d and 51st Field Hospitals, and five subdepots in the blood distribution system: the 406th, 528th, and 946th Mobile Medical Laboratories at Nha Trang, Qui Nhon, and Long Binh, respectively; the Naval Support Activity Hospital, Da Nang; and the 96th Evacuation Hospital, Vung Tau.

As troop strength grew and combat casualties increased, the task of distributing whole blood, plasma, and related products in South Vietnam developed into the largest blood distribution system ever undertaken by a single organization.

Colonel James E. McCarty, MC, became Blood Program Officer, PACOM, in June 1968 and commander of the 406th in Japan at the same time. He and his predecessor, Colonel Metzger, visited South Vietnam regularly, conferred with the surgeon, and inspected blood facilities throughout the country.

Initial Sources of Whole Blood

The primary source for whole blood used in South Vietnam until July 1966 was the 406th Medical Laboratory in Japan. Mobile bleeding teams were dispatched from the laboratory to donor resources in Japan, Korea, Okinawa, and Taiwan. A very valuable donor resource was found in the Yokosuka Naval Base when the Pacific fleet came in, and reserve donor resources also existed in Hawaii, Guam, and the Philippines. With vigorous command support and the dedicated work of blood-drawing teams, supply kept pace with demand until June 1966. Blood collections in PACOM rose from 201 units in January 1965 to 7,426 in January 1966 and 12,984 in June 1966.

Blood collected in PACOM was processed and shipped from the 406th in Japan to large troop concentrations along the coast of South

Vietnam at Saigon, Nha Trang, Qui Nhon, and Da Nang. By 1965, it was apparent that this plan would not work because aircraft could not be scheduled economically from Japan to each of the four areas regularly enough to keep the supply levels of blood at the proper level. Communications between Japan and the coastal cities were poor, and shipments of blood often arrived in Vietnam without the knowledge of those persons handling it. Planners had also become sharply aware that blood could not be handled as a routine supply item even in a dedicated medical supply system.

In short, by 1965 it was clear in PACOM that the whole blood distribution system should consist of a central depot in Saigon with several small mobile subdepots located in areas of high troop intensity.

Agencies for Expansion of Blood Supply

The Military Blood Program Agency

In June 1966, the need for whole blood in Vietnam became urgent. Blood donor resources in PACOM had been exceeded, and the blood program officer estimated that 1,000 units of low titer group O blood per week would be needed. CINCUSARPAC sent a request to the MBPA (Military Blood Program Agency) to ship the needed blood to the 406th.

Four years earlier, in May 1962, responsibility for implementing and co-ordinating the whole blood program in CONUS was delegated to the Secretary of the Army by the Secretary of Defense. Hence, The Surgeon General of the Army established the MBPA on 17 July 1962 to support emergency requirements for whole blood in war. The agency, staffed by medical officers of the three services, maintained close working relationships with the U.S. Public Health Service, the Office of Emergency Planning, Executive Office of the President, and the American Red Cross.

Armed Services Whole Blood Processing Laboratory

The MBPA incorporated the donor collection and processing capabilities of the three military departments. Blood was collected by 42 donor centers designated by The Surgeons General of the Army, Navy, and Air Force and shipped by air to the triservice ASWBPL (Armed Services Whole Blood Processing Laboratory), McGuire Air Force Base. (*Chart 13*) All group O blood was titered, and after a thorough inspection and verification of groups, Rh types, and other essentials, blood was flown via Elmendorf Air Force Base, Alaska, to Yokota Air Force Base in Japan. At each point, shipments were re-iced, if necessary, and flown to the 406th Medical Laboratory in Japan. From Japan, whole blood was

CHART 13—MILITARY BLOOD PROGRAM AGENCY OPERATIONAL SCHEME FOR TRISERVICE COLLECTING-PROCESSING OF WHOLE BLOOD TO SHIP THROUGH THE ARMED SERVICES PROCESSING LABORATORY, MCGUIRE AIR FORCE BASE, N.J., 1966–70

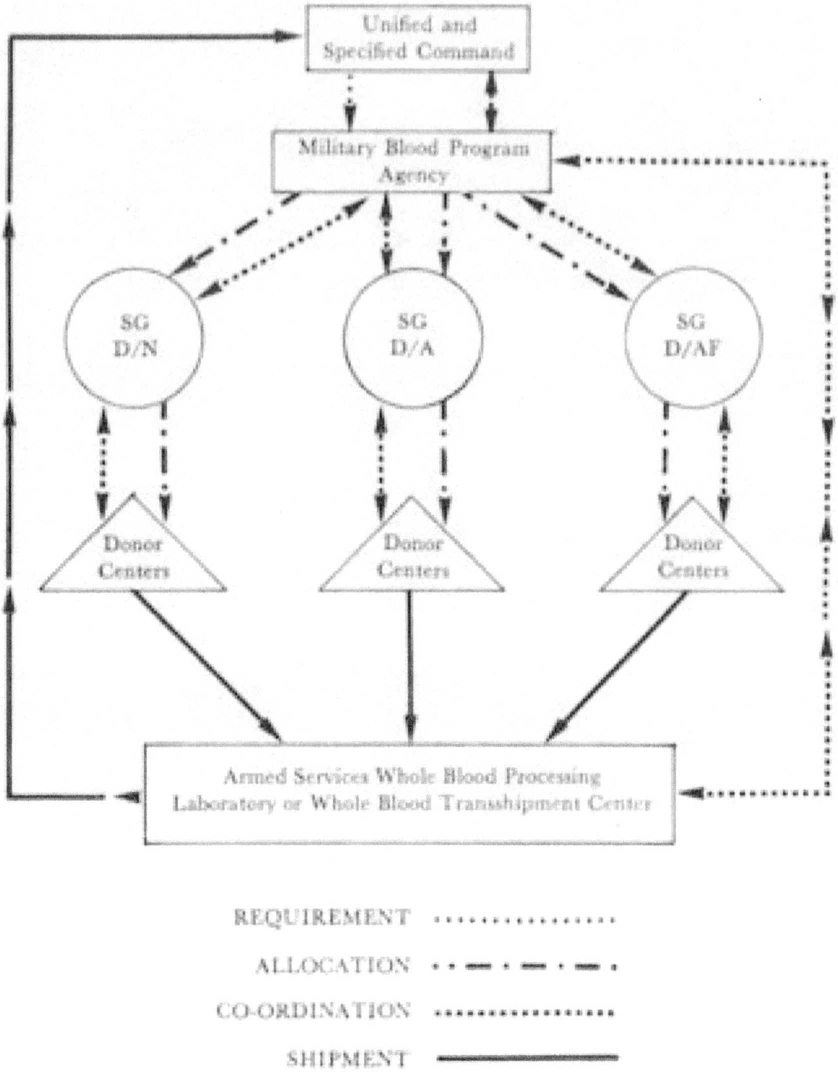

flown to the 9th Medical Laboratory, Saigon, and distributed from there to subdepots in South Vietnam.

The first shipment of whole blood, 2,036 units, arrived in Japan from the United States in July 1966.

From July 1966 to 1967, two shipments of 1,500 to 2,500 units of whole blood were received from CONUS each week. To boost blood needs, Colonel Metzger recommended in 1967 that daily shipments to total 5,000 units each week be made from CONUS to arrive in Japan early in the morning, from Mondays through Fridays. Daily shipments began in mid-August 1967. The total number of units of blood collected and shipped to Vietnam are shown in Table 9.

Table 9.—Number of Units of Blood Collected and Shipped, by Year, to the Central Blood Bank in Vietnam by the 406th Medical Laboratory, U.S. Army, Japan

Year	Units collected [1]	Units shipped
	Number	Number
1966	130, 308	115, 869
1967	222, 534	213, 022
1968	399, 724	351, 519
1969	385, 883	348, 409
1970 [2]	73, 109	59, 175
Total	1, 211, 558	1, 087, 994

[1] The total figures for each year include blood shipped to the 406th Medical Laboratory in Japan by CONUS and that collected in PACOM by the 406th.

[2] Excludes blood collected and shipped in December 1970. December statistics were not available.

Source: Report, Administrative Division, 406th Medical Laboratory, USAMC, Japan, 1970.

From 1969, whole blood was flown by MATS C–141 Starlifter to Japan. This blood, plus fresh frozen plasma and whole blood obtained by the 406th, was flown by commercial airline to the USARV Central Blood Bank in Saigon and after June 1969 to Cam Ranh Bay, the new location of the blood bank. (*Map 5*) Blood was approximately 7 days old by this time. Most of it went forward by C–130 fixed wing aircraft to one of the six subdepots at Long Binh, Nha Trang, Qui Nhon, Pleiku, Chu Lai, and Da Nang. From these subdepots, blood of all types and fresh frozen plasma were sent by fixed wing aircraft, helicopter, or ambulance to the various field, evacuation, and surgical hospitals. Low titer group

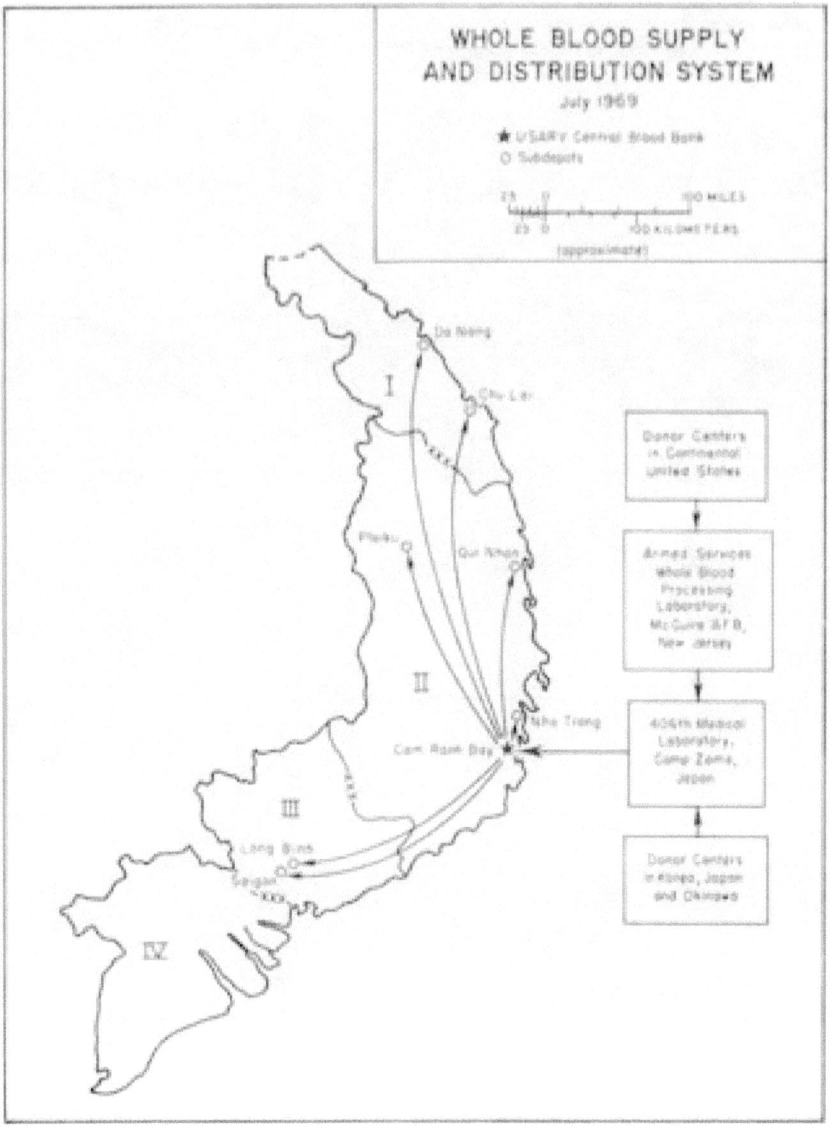

Map 5

O positive blood was shipped from the subdepots to division clearing stations by helicopter.

The Department of Defense, and thus MBPA, felt that blood quotas should be assigned according to available donor resources. The military departments originally felt that quotas should be assigned according to

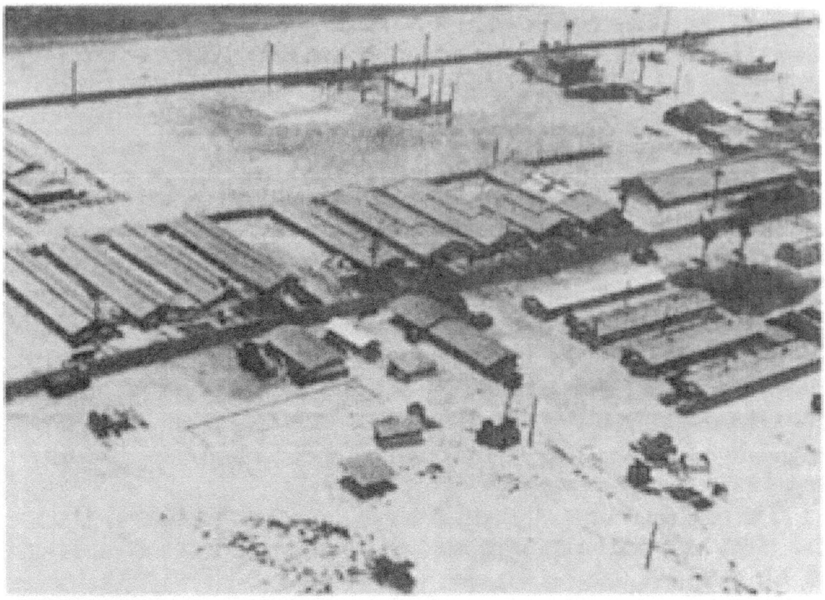

An Overview of the New Central Blood Bank at Cam Ranh Bay, June 1969

their blood requirements. Fortunately, this problem was resolved early and essentially the following distribution prevailed:

Agency	Army	Air Force	Navy
MBPA (recommendations)............percent..	50	30	20
Military departments (furnished).......percent..	51	29	20

Relocation of the Central Blood Bank

After the Tet Offensive in 1968, military officials feared that another such offensive would interrupt the supply of blood from the USARV Central Blood Bank in Saigon, or that the airfield at Tan Son Nhut might be seized. Plans were initiated to construct a new central blood bank at Cam Ranh Bay on the grounds of the 6th Convalescent Center. The new laboratory was completed in June 1969 and the USARV Central Blood Bank moved there in July 1969.

The building, with 1,000 square feet of laboratory floor space and 600 square feet of cement under cover, accommodated a 1,800 cubic foot walk-in refrigerator. The neat new structure was considered to be in a more secure area at Cam Ranh Bay than in Saigon, and air transportation from Japan was readily available. (*See Map 5.*) Maximum flexibility was achieved by the relocation of the central blood bank. The

3d Field Hospital, redesignated a subdepot, could quickly revert to a central blood bank if an emergency arose, and the subdepot at Da Nang, after expansion, was fully capable of serving as a central blood bank.

Group and Type-Specific Blood

In early 1965, it was decided that only universal donor low titer group O blood would be shipped to Vietnam, and that the use of group and type-specific blood would be confined to the offshore hospitals in Japan and in the Philippines. The great advantage of universal donor blood is that it is impossible to give a patient the wrong group of blood. As the requirements for blood increased, and as hospitals in Vietnam became more sophisticated, blood program officials decided to utilize fully the available donor population. Less than 45 percent of the donor population had group O low titer blood, and 55 percent of the donor population was not being bled.

The first shipments of group A blood arrived in Vietnam in December 1965, and shipments with random blood group distribution, groups A, AB, B, and O, without selection, arrived in January 1966. The clearing companies and forward surgical hospitals continued to use only group O low titer blood because they could not cross match, but evacuation hospitals began to give other type-specific transfusions almost exclusively.

Unfortunately, random shipments resulted in excessive amounts of group A blood in the depots in Vietnam. With the institution of shipments from CONUS by MBPA in July 1966, the numbers of units of universal donor group O low titer blood shipped to Vietnam increased, and by 1967, shipments exceeded requirements by 65 percent. As more and more Vietnamese were cared for in U.S. military hospitals, with the Vietnamization of the combat role, a new problem with blood group distribution arose. The requirements for group B increased in proportion to the number of Vietnamese admitted to American military hospitals. The approximate percentage blood group distribution for American and Vietnamese populations in the following tabulation readily show that Vietnamese required more group B blood:

	Specific blood types			
	A	*AB*	*B*	*O*
American troops . . . . percent . .	39	3	14	44
Vietnamese troops . . . . percent . .	21	6	31	42

Transfusion Reactions

Hemolytic and Nonhemolytic Transfusion Reactions

Between March 1967 and June 1969, approximately 364,900 transfusions were recorded. During that period, 38 hemolytic and 979 nonhemolytic transfusion reactions were reported, or about 1 hemolytic transfusion reaction per 9,600 transfusions and one nonhemolytic reaction per 370 transfusions. Causes of the nonhemolytic reactions are unknown and while they never threatened life, these reactions were considered detrimental to the well-being of the severely wounded patient. The cause of these reactions is exceedingly complex, and much research is needed in this neglected field.

The Coagulopathies

Bleeding problems, called variously the oozing syndrome, tomato juice syndrome, or red ink syndrome, were frightening to the most experienced battle surgeon. To see a patient suddenly begin to bleed profusely from every orifice and wound just as heroic surgery appeared to be successful was a dramatic experience.

Coagulopathies may be divided into two groups, if it is remembered that the division is an oversimplification. Since coagulopathies usually occur in combinations and rarely in the pure form, study under field conditions is almost impossible. Coagulopathies that respond well to fresh blood are attributed to deficiencies of platelets or deficiencies of coagulation principles other than platelets. The latter principles respond well to fresh frozen plasma or fresh blood. Coagulopathies that do not respond well to fresh blood may be attributed to circulating anticoagulants, disseminated intravascular coagulation, or circulating intravascular fibrinolysins.

While physicians generally recognized the classification of coagulopathies, there was little agreement about the proper treatment. One group of physicians treated all coagulation problems with fresh blood while others differentiated the various syndromes and used more specific treatments, such as fresh blood, fresh frozen plasma, cortisone, heparin, epsilon, aminocaproic acid—or prayer. Fortunately the number of patients suffering from coagulation problems was small, but the threat after massive transfusions and surgery was ever present.

Fresh Frozen Plasma

In April 1968, fresh frozen plasma was introduced in Vietnam as a means for controlling coagulopathies following surgery and massive transfusions. The availability of fresh frozen plasma resulted in a decrease in the quantity of fresh whole blood drawn in Vietnam. Fresh plasma is obtained at the 406th Medical Laboratory in Japan by the process of plasmapheresis from a limited group of donors of the AB group—the ideal donors for fresh plasma. These donors may be bled every week or every other week. Blood from them is spun down, plasma rises to the top, and red cells settle at the bottom. While plasma is drawn off in satellite bags and frozen immediately, red cells are returned to the donor.

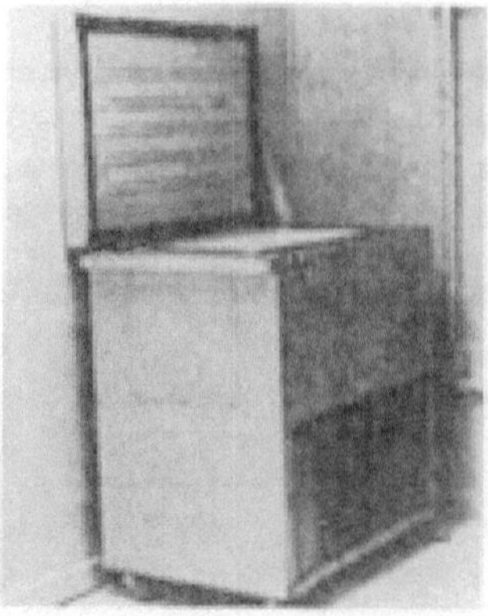

A 2.5-Cubic Foot Freezer in Which Fresh Frozen Plasma Is Stored

Since plasma proteins are replenished rapidly, each donor may contribute 2 units weekly for as long as 2 years without effects.

Donors in the AB group have no isoantibodies in their plasma and it may be given to patients of any blood type—a real breakthrough.

Wastage of Blood

The amount of whole blood outdated because it was not used in 21 days was frequently significant and occasionally, during lulls in the fighting, reached 50 percent of the blood in Vietnam per month. The average amount of outdating was approximately 29 percent with extremes of 9 percent and 50 percent.

Use of whole blood was best during periods of greatest military activity. While much speculation and discussion transpired about this significant problem, the simple facts are that blood was usually from 4 to 7 days old before it arrived in Vietnam. Outdating was difficult to eliminate because filling requisitions instantly for subdepots throughout Vietnam was impossible. Some waste of blood was the price that had to be paid to assure that not one fighting man would die for the want of blood.

Most blood 21 to 31 days old was shipped to ARVN hospitals for local use and for Free World forces if they desired it. During the early days of the buildup, 31-day-old blood was destroyed, but as the war progressed, blood was converted to plasma lyophilized by the vacuum system.

Technical Research and Innovations

Lengthening the Life of Blood

Efforts were constantly made to extend the shelf life of blood. One of the most promising was the addition of small amounts of the amino acid adenine which increased the shelf life of whole blood to 40 days. Blood with such an additive was tried on a limited basis in Vietnam during 1969. The blood was transfused to patients admitted to the hospitals at Long Binh, and no adverse effects were found in numbers of clinical tests. As soon as the oxygen-carrying capacity of adenine-treated red cells can be improved, adenine may well be added to all units of liquid preserved blood used in combat military blood banking. Experiments indicate that the oxygen-carrying capacity of treated red cells may be increased by adding small amounts of inosine.

Freezers for Fresh Frozen Plasma

The freezing compartment of an ordinary refrigerator is not cold enough to keep fresh frozen plasma for more than a week or two. Factor V, the most critical of all clotting factors, is present in the plasma, and it deteriorates slowly at temperatures above $-20°C$. A small freezer, used by construction engineers to cool steel rivets, was ideal for storing fresh frozen plasma. Steel rivets contract when cooled and expand to give a snug fit as they warm up. After diligent searching, enough of these freezers were found for all hospitals in Vietnam. By July 1969, a newly designed 4-cubic foot freezer, similar to the construction engineer's freezer, was issued in Vietnam.

The Styrofoam Blood Box

While the war in South Vietnam will be remembered by most military men as the war in which air mobility came of age, it will be remembered by many people, both Vietnamese and American, as the war of the white styrofoam blood box. The styrofoam blood box was introduced in late 1965 and was without question one of the most important technical advancements to come out of the blood distribution program. Major William S. Collins II, director of the blood bank at the 406th Medical Laboratory, suggested modifying the standard disposable blood box by replacing the cardboard divide insert with a styrofoam insert which he had devised. The new insert, when placed in a cardboard shipping container, permitted shipment of blood at the required temperature regardless of outside temperatures. The shipping container is easier to handle and was less susceptible to damage or destruction. Major Collins received $935 for his suggestion, and his innovation resulted in a first-year savings of $56,000 and a new flexibility in military blood banking.

The Collins box, which occupies only 3 cubic feet and weighs only 40 pounds when filled with 18 units of whole blood and wet ice, replaced the Hollinger box which occupies 8 cubic feet and weighs 115 pounds when filled with 24 units of blood and wet ice. In addition to weighing less, the Collins box offers other equally important advantages: it costs only $1.40, or $98.60 less than the $100 Hollinger box; it is expendable and does not have to be returned through the system to Japan. The Collins box maintains an adequate ice level for 48 hours, twice as long as the Hollinger box. The castoff Collins styrofoam blood boxes were grabbed by American servicemen and Vietnamese civilians to be used as private iceboxes in hot and dusty Vietnam.

Significant Problems

Wet icemaking machines used to manufacture ice for blood shipments plagued their users at all blood depots with maintenance problems. Research to resolve the problem was started by the USARV blood program officer.

Another significant question concerned how much universal donor group O low titer whole blood could be given to a casualty before he would have a reaction to his hereditary specific type and group. At least one important experiment was done at Walter Reed Army Medical Center on a small group of men who had received from 21 to 44 units of universal donor group O blood, but results were inconclusive.

The Donor System

For the first time in U.S. military history, every unit of whole blood used to support the war was donated free of charge by military personnel, their dependents, and civilians employed at military installations.

Donors were not motivated by profit. No high-pressure advertising programs were permitted, yet nearly a million and a half volunteers gave blood. Not once was it necessary to initiate contracts for blood to be supplied by the American Red Cross or the American Association of Blood Banks. Even in the most difficult times, when blood requirements reached 38,000 units a month, the civilian blood collection system was not upset by the additional military requirements to support an ongoing war.

Most of the credit for donor recruitment must go to the young officers and the sergeants. These dedicated individuals instilled such confidence in their men that the fear of giving blood and the social pressures against the war were overcome.

CHAPTER X

Medical Research

Initial Efforts in Southeast Asia

In July 1962, a group from WRAIR was sent to Southeast Asia to evaluate the existing resources for medical research and to develop plans for co-ordination and expansion. They surveyed the laboratories then operating in East and Southeast Asia: the Air Force's Fifth Epidemiological Flight at Yamata, Japan, with one air-transportable trailer-type bacteriology laboratory, the 406th Medical General Laboratory at Camp Zama, Japan, the NAMRU-2 (U.S. Naval Medical Research Unit No. 2) in Taipei, Taiwan, the U.S. Army Medical Research Unit in Kuala Lumpur, Malaysia, and the U.S. Army Medical Component of the SEATO (Southeast Asia Treaty Organization) Medical Research Laboratory in Thailand.

At the completion of their survey, the study group recommended expansion of the existing medical research program to include studies of U.S. troops and of local national troops and civilian populations, allocation of additional personnel and funds, and establishment in Saigon of a WRAIR medical research unit, similar to those in Bangkok and Kuala Lumpur, because a theater laboratory would not be able to deal with all the subjects to be covered in the expanded program.

In November 1963, as a result of the survey group's recommendations, Lieutenant Colonel (later Colonel) Paul E. Teschan, MC, was sent to Vietnam with a team of seven officers and 12 enlisted men. They quickly established liaison with United States and Vietnamese military medical staffs and installations, with the Public Health Division of USOM (U.S. Operations Mission), AID, and, through them, with the Minister of Health, members of the Pasteur Institute, the medical school faculties, medical missionaries, and representatives of private U.S. charitable and medical foundations. They thus had access to all populations—Vietnamese and American, military and civilian—that was required to detect problems and settings in which productive investigation could be done and to deploy and support qualified investigators.

Studies of the Medical Research Team

Initially the team studied infectious disease, combat surgery, and military psychiatry, and evaluated new medical materiel. Their first effort was a serologic survey among U.S. military advisers in the Delta region for evidence of viral hepatitis, leptospirosis, and dengue-related viruses.

Cholera

Cholera, absent from Vietnam for 10 years, spread from Cambodia into Saigon-Cho Lon and some provinces. Several thousand cases appeared within about 2 months, and the clinics and hospitals were soon overwhelmed. The disease was found among the destitute and frequently in immunized persons. Cholera rarely appeared in more than one member of a family and generally ran a self-limited course, perhaps somewhat shortened by antibiotics. No Americans were affected.

Dr. Richard Finkelstein, from WRAIR, and Dr. Howard Noyes, from the SEATO laboratory in Bangkok, went to Saigon to work in the Pasteur Institute. Captain Robert A. Phillips, MC, USN, and the staff of NAMRU–2 arrived from Taipei, instituted their mass treatment system of replacement of massive fluid and electrolyte losses, quickly taught it to the Vietnamese, and soon virtually eliminated further deaths from cholera.

Plague

Plague caused concern as a potential threat to U.S. troops. Darkened streets were alive with rats, and the rats were alive with fleas. In late 1962, during a plague epidemic in Saigon, Colonel (later Brigadier General) William D. Tigertt, MC, and Lieutenant Colonel Kevin G. Barry, MC, had established a small research unit with personnel from the 7th Medical Laboratory, whose efforts were directed primarily toward plague surveillance and diagnosis. Later, the liaison already developed during the cholera epidemic led to the joint study of plague by the Ministry of Health, the Pasteur Institute, and the WRAIR team. Colonel Teschan was appointed by the Minister of Health to the reactivated Commission for Pathologic Researches in Vietnam. Such common enterprise was later extended to studies of hemorrhagic dengue which produced hemorrhagic fever in Vietnamese children and also affected U.S. troops.

During its second year, under the direction of Lieutenant Colonel Stefano Vivona, MC, the team developed a close relationship with the Pasteur Institute in Saigon; through this collaborative effort, the only plague research laboratory in Southeast Asia was constructed and operated. From this laboratory, the extent and severity of plague in Vietnam were documented; for example, whereas only eight cases were reported from a single province in 1961, by 1966 human plague was shown to be present in every province in I, II, and III Corps areas, and in one province in IV Corps area, with 4,500 cases occurring in 1965 alone. Studies of rodent reservoirs and flea vectors of plague revealed new endemic foci, and during a pilot program for rodent and vector control in the Minh Mang district of Cho Lon, rat fleas were found to be resistant to DDT. These data, in addition to laboratory studies of the insecticides dieldrin and Diazinon, provided the Ministry of Health with information essential for reducing the vectors and controlling the disease.

The common house shrew was shown for the first time to be a reservoir of plague; an asymptomatic carrier state of virulent plague bacilli in the throats of healthy people was demonstrated for the first time in Vietnam; rat and flea survey programs and insecticide evaluation programs were expanded; and a program was initiated for production and evaluation of a lyophilized, attenuated living plague vaccine.

Malaria

During its third year, 1965–66, under the direction of Lieutenant Colonel (later Colonel) Robert J. T. Joy, MC, the medical research team expanded its mission to include specific research studies by individual team members, support of other research studies by outside investigators, and collection of medical information or health data for WRAIR, which would serve as a guide for research in the laboratories of the USAMRDC (U.S. Army Medical Research and Development Command). Specific areas of interest included malaria, plague, gastrointestinal disease, fevers of undetermined origin, combat psychiatry, environmental stress, and other causes of morbidity and mortality in U.S. soldiers.

The data collected warned the team of the possibility of a rise in the number of cases of chloroquine-resistant falciparum malaria and they devoted much of their effort to this disease. Among their contributions were the discovery of asymptomatic malaria, with its potential for importation to the continental United States; documentation of failures of malaria discipline and personal protective measures, which provided information needed for control; introduction of new therapeutic drugs (Fanasil and pyrimethamine) and other regimens for the treatment of malaria; and provision of consultative advice to the various command surgeons. A major contribution to the control of malaria in Vietnam was the introduction of DDS (diaminodiphenylsulfone). The efficacy of this drug as a prophylactic agent was confirmed in volunteers in the United States, and in 1966, a field test in Vietnam proved its value in combat troops. Subsequently, it was routinely used by military personnel in Vietnam for prophylaxis against falciparum malaria.

The team recommended that a central rehabilitation hospital for malaria patients be established and used simultaneously as a center for studying the disease and the evaluation of new therapeutic agents. This hospital was approved by The Surgeon General and became the 6th Convalescent Center at Cam Ranh Bay. A formal link with the Navy preventive medicine unit in Da Nang provided for the collection of specimens by the Navy unit, with laboratory support from the team, and for the exchange of information and research data. The 61st Medical Detachment of the 20th Preventive Medicine Unit (entomology) was established and worked with the team in the laboratory.

In the fall of 1966, the team in essence drafted a USARV regulation on malaria control guided by letters and comments from Colonel Tigertt; a medical research team for malaria survey for USARV was established; and Captain Anthony T. C. Bourke, MC, was appointed the USARV consultant in malaria.

Stress

Studies done by the medical research team of neuroendocrine stress caused by combat, in helicopter crewmen and Special Forces "A" Detachment members, contributed significantly to the understanding of the pathophysiology of stress in the soldier. Studies of heat stress incurred by crews of the Mohawk (OV–1) aircraft led to changes in clothing and to ventilation of the cockpit, measures which materially improved crew comfort and efficiency. Collaborative studies with the Department of Neuropsychiatry of the ARVN Cong Hoa Hospital led to a better understanding of the stresses of combat affecting both American and Vietnamese soldiers.

Fever of Undetermined Origin

A major collaborative study done by the team with the 93d Evacuation Hospital and the SEATO laboratory in Bangkok resulted in determining the specific etiology of FUO in 60 percent of patients studied. Of the cases diagnosed, 50 percent were due to dengue, with Chikungunya, scrub typhus, and malaria accounting for most of the remainder. These laboratory results, carefully correlated with clinical findings, enabled clinicians to suspect these diseases, in the absence of classical findings, early in the course of hospitalization.

Renal Failure

In February 1966, Colonel Barry arrived at the 3d Field Hospital in Saigon to institute clinical research studies in patients with malaria, including studies of body water, extracellular fluid, blood volume, and renal function. Because the only facilities for performing hemodialysis were in Japan and the Philippines, delays in evacuation and treatment of patients with acute renal failure often resulted in increased morbidity and mortality. Colonel Barry, recognizing the need for in-country treatment of this complication, established the first renal unit in Vietnam at the 3d Field Hospital.

Special Projects

The Field Epidemiologic Survey Team

The war in Vietnam pointed up deficiencies in the knowledge of certain important tropical diseases and, more significantly, the deficiencies in the ability to predict noneffectiveness and in the application of preventive techniques. It also provided the opportunity for a unique and valuable experiment in medical support of military operations in a hostile environment.

The FEST (Field Epidemiologic Survey Team) was organized in May 1966 by Lieutenant Colonel Llewellyn J. Legters, MC, preventive medicine officer of the USA John F. Kennedy Center for Special Warfare at Fort Bragg, N.C., who recognized that a research group operating in the remote areas where U.S. military forces were being committed could study the epidemiology of tropical diseases in the environment where most of them were transmitted.

The FEST, composed of Special Forces officers and enlisted technicians stationed at Fort Bragg, was trained at Fort Bragg and at WRAIR in specific laboratory and field epidemiological skills suitable for studying diseases of special interest to the Army Medical Department and in providing medical support, preventive and curative, to ground troops in Vietnam. Training was oriented primarily to specified scientific areas of interest such as the entomological aspects of tropical sprue, febrile illness, schistosomiasis, filariasis, dengue, and malaria.

After the training period, FEST was formally constituted as an element of WRAIR, deployed to Vietnam on 26 September 1966, and became part of the medical research team in Saigon for administration and logistics, but was attached to Headquarters, 5th Special Forces Group.

The studies of this team which continued through 1968, diminishing as the war became conventionalized, generated valuable scientific information about malaria, plague, schistosomiasis, filariasis, tropical sprue, and other ailments.

Dermatological Research

The character of warfare in Vietnam also created unique opportunities for research on cutaneous diseases of military importance. At the height of the rainy season, the rates of disabling skin disease among infantrymen were extremely high, reaching 50 percent in some rifle companies. Surgeons at the infantry battalion level were often overwhelmed by the number of soldiers displaying skin lesions of uncertain etiology which were slow to heal despite vigorous topical and systemic antibiotic therapy. Combat commanders and physicians alike became extremely receptive to scientific investigations of the common skin diseases that had defied the most heroic efforts at prevention and control.

The U.S. Army Medical Research and Development Command sent a special field epidemiological research team from WRAIR to the Mekong Delta in 1968. The team had trained in simulated tropical combat environment at camps in the southern United States and in the Florida Everglades under the supervision of Dr. Harvey Blank of the University of Miami (Fla.) School of Medicine. Mr. David Taplin, also a member of the University of Miami faculty, conducted workshops in applied microbiology and subsequently accompanied the team to Vietnam to help establish a base laboratory.

The reception accorded the team assured them of the support so necessary for productive research under wartime conditions. The commanding general of the 9th Infantry Division, Major General (later Lieutenant General) Julian J. Ewell, pledged the full co-operation of his officers and men. The requirement for a laboratory in the Delta was more than met when the USARV surgeon, General Neel, made available a completely equipped MUST unit that provided an ideal setting for microbiological studies, with negligible risks of contamination from mud, dust, and insect life. Colonel William A. Akers, MC, Chief, Dermatology Research Unit, Letterman Army Institute of Research, promised co-operation and provided personal liaison at theater and division levels in Vietnam. Most important of all was the complete acceptance of the team by the officers and men of combat units who displayed a cheerful willingness to be examined, despite the incursions on their limited free time.

Under the leadership of Captain (later Major) Alfred M. Allen, MC, the team conducted intensive research among combat forces, support troops, and neighboring Vietnamese populations in the Delta. They examined American and Vietnamese infantrymen at forward company and battalion areas in active fire zones and accompanied infantry units on patrol to evaluate proposed methods of skin disease prevention. Use of portable field laboratories and special culture media permitted isolation of pathogens that had eluded detection by standard methods. In less than 6 months, Captain Allen's team had precisely identified the populations most likely to develop common disabling skin diseases, isolated the offending pathogens, measured the effects of exposure, and initiated effective new methods of prevention and treatment.

The chief causes of cutaneous disability in American combat forces were inflammatory ringworm, ecthymatous pyoderma, and tropical immersion foot. Disease rates correlated with the degree of exposure to such things as insect bites and prolonged contact with wet clothing. Prickly heat, acne vulgaris, and tinea versicolor, while common, as a general rule were not disabling, nor was cystic (tropical) acne, which can be very disabling, a significant cause of manpower loss.

Elastase-producing fungi were found to be the major cause of inflammatory ringworm in the American combat forces. The usual athlete's foot type was surprisingly rare, being replaced by intensely inflamed, serum-oozing lesions on the dorsa of the feet, the ankles, and groin, often forming multiple small abscesses in hair follicles. The clinical features and the microbiological characteristics of the disease indicated that the infections were transmitted by a source in Vietnam rather than by irritation of old, latent infections, as previously believed. A search for sources of infection revealed that 25 percent of the wild rats tested were infected with organisms which were morphologically indistinguishable from those recovered from American soldiers.

In contrast to those found in infantrymen, the infections among support troops strongly resembled the type found among troops in training at southern United States military bases during the summer.

Penicillin treatment significantly reduced healing time of ecthymatous pyodermas in American soldiers despite a prevalence of penicillin-resistant staphylococci. Erythromycin was also effective in a small number of cases. Tetracycline was avoided because of the high proportion of resistant streptococci recovered from the pyodermas.

The clinical and pathological features of tropical immersion foot were consistent with low-grade cold injury. Soldiers who had contracted the condition following prolonged immersion displayed increased susceptibility to repeat injury even after complete healing had occurred. Skin biopsies showed chronic inflammation and dilatation of vascular channels.

Skin infections in Vietnamese adults were strikingly different from those among Americans, even in military populations with identical exposure. *Trichophyton mentagrophytes* infections and streptococcal pyoderma were rare; ringworm, although fairly common, was nearly always caused by an atypical variant of *Trichophyton rubrum* which produced a chronic, scaly, dry rash generally confined to the waist. Vietnamese children, on the other hand, were similar to American combat troops in their frequent experience with streptococcal pyoderma and ringworm.

After Captain Allen's departure from Vietnam, dermatological research was continued by Captain Joseph Thompson, MC, Captain Joseph M. Ballo, MC, and Lieutenant Colonel Robert T. Cutting, MC. The results of two field trials to determine the efficacy of griseofulvin in the prevention of ringworm infection showed that it was significantly protective, provided the recommended dosage schedule was strictly observed.

The field dermatology research program in Vietnam was rewarding in the relatively brief span of its existence. Early application of the measures recommended on the basis of the team's findings dramatically lowered disability rates wherever they were put into effect. Research priorities were realigned to be more directly aimed at prevention of those diseases having the greatest impact on combat manpower. Laboratories in the United States focused their attention on the newly found clues to pathogenesis of the common disabling skin infections. Representative isolates of pathogenic strains of fungi and bacteria recovered in Vietnam were collected for future study. The influence of the research findings even extended to the development of new items of tropical military footwear. As a direct result of the dedicated efforts of this team, and because of military-civilian co-operation, development of effective methods to prevent the devastating effects of skin diseases came, for the first time, within reach.

Photographic Coverage of Army Medical Activities

During the latter part of 1965 it became evident that photographic coverage of Army medical activities in Vietnam was unsatisfactory. Since the Medical Audiovisual Department, WRAIR, was capable of providing highly professional still and motion picture support of the WRAIR's diverse research activities, it was decided to field a photography team to be attached to the WRAIR research team but to be equally responsive to direction from the USARV surgeon.

Two weeks after the decision was made, four civilian volunteers, all from WRAIR, began a comprehensive coverage of surgery, helicopter evacuation, combat "medics" in action, field hospital operations, and other medical activities wherever and whenever they saw them. They formed a highly mobile and aggressive team, not only responding to requests and direction from the medical command, but also seeking out on their own initiative areas and activities requiring photographic coverage

The Surgeon General, realizing that the team approach was the most efficient means of acquiring accurate and timely pictorial records of the Army's medical effort in Vietnam, directed that additional personnel and funds be provided to establish a permanent team of military medical photographers. This team, consisting of one officer, one noncommissioned officer, and three enlisted men, became operational in December 1967. Adhering to the pattern already established, the new group continued to work closely with the USARV medical and surgical consultants, following the action to the areas of greatest activity. Thus began the collection of thousands of color slides and hundreds of thousands of feet of motion picture film which later became the basis for film libraries, not only in the United States (such as those at WRAIR and at the Medical Field Service School at Fort Sam Houston), but also in Europe, Hawaii, and Asia. At least three major film productions resulted from the footage obtained, one on helicopter evacuation, another on MUST, and a third, the award-winning "Army Medicine in Vietnam."

Surgical Research

In its fourth year, the team concentrated on surgical research and on testing the FEST concept. The research was done by a group which was attached to the team in April 1966, initially at the 93d Evacuation Hospital, later at the 3d Surgical Hospital, and finally at the 24th Evacuation Hospital. The group demonstrated that studies of the type conducted in "shock units" in the United States can be carried out with satisfactory results on combat casualties in the field. Later studies conducted by the research group contributed to the knowledge of many other subjects.

Recognition of the seriousness of pulmonary insufficiency in shock, particularly in patients with nonthoracic injuries, led to extensive research in the management of this complication. Plans were made for the development and testing of new respiratory assistance devices.

Further progress was made in the development and use of plastic polymers as tissue adhesives in controlling bleeding and repairing internal organs. Spray guns containing the adhesive were provided the surgical research team for use in treating casualties in Vietnam.

New methods for fixation of fractures of the jaw were studied, as was a new technique using a silicone plastic placed directly into oral wounds to restore temporary oral integrity until reconstructive surgery could be performed.

Other innovations under study by the research group were the use of electrical anesthesia, laser irradiation, synthetic blood vessels, plasma expanders and new additives in the preservation of whole blood, Sulfamylon ointment for control of infection in burns, and various methods for suppression of an immune response of the body to homografts and transplants.

CHAPTER XI

Laboratory Support

Evolution of the System

The development of the medical laboratory system in Vietnam derived from knowledge and experience from the Far East Medical Research Unit attached to the 406th Medical General Laboratory in Japan, the U.S. Army Medical Research Unit (Malaya), the U.S. Component of the SEATO Medical Laboratory in Bangkok, and the Field Medical Laboratory Project, USARMDC. The system was based on a concept of the laboratory as a component of medical service, with a specific function of generating medical technical information for the purpose of patient care, disease prevention, advice to the command, and forensic activity.

The first medical laboratory unit in Vietnam, a mobile detachment of the 406th Medical General Laboratory, began operations as laboratory augmentation of the 8th Field Hospital in Nha Trang in 1962.

In late 1965, the 528th and 946th Mobile Laboratories of the 9th Medical Laboratory arrived in Vietnam and were placed under operational control of the 406th Mobile Laboratory. These units were to support the 85th and 93d Evacuation Hospitals. Within 6 months, the headquarters and base section of the 9th Medical Laboratory arrived and assumed control over these units. In August 1967, the 406th Mobile Laboratory was placed under operational control of the 9th Medical Laboratory.

In January 1968, the 74th Medical Laboratory was activated and organized to replace the 406th Medical Laboratory (Mobile) and was placed under operational control of the 9th Medical Laboratory. By September 1968, the 946th and 528th Medical Laboratories (Mobile) were inactivated and their personnel assigned to the 9th Medical Laboratory. These two mobile laboratories, or mobile sections of the 9th Medical Laboratory, continued operations in Long Binh and Qui Nhon.

The 9th Medical Laboratory

From May to December 1966, the 9th Medical Laboratory was assigned to the 44th Medical Brigade under the 1st Logistical Command. The equipment was antique, and efforts to obtain new equipment and supplies were unrewarding. Building facilities, located 15 feet from a dirt highway, were inappropriate and inadequate. As a result, little productive work was accomplished considering the high potential of the personnel. In December 1966, the laboratory moved from the small dusty store to a newer building, a Vietnamese constructed barracks. Although the building was larger, the site was less favorable.

In June 1967, authorities decided to construct new facilities for the central laboratories at Long Binh for the purpose of establishing more appropriate buildings, bringing the 9th Medical Laboratory and the 20th Preventive Medicine Unit together for more co-ordinated function, bringing the 9th Medical Laboratory in close support of major hospitals at Long Binh to free a mobile laboratory for service elsewhere, and bringing the 9th Medical Laboratory in close range of its supply and personnel support units. It was not until December 1968, however, that the laboratory moved into its new fixed facilities, but not before it had been exposed to hostile fire and isolated twice earlier that year.

The 44th Medical Brigade was transferred from 1st Logistical Command to the Surgeon, USARV, in 1967. After this transfer, a set of equipment and supplies, developed by a USAMRDC contract, was ordered from manufacturers in sufficient quantities to provide for all medical laboratory services within the 44th Medical Brigade.

In his role as USARV pathology consultant, Colonel Baker recommended assignments of all medical laboratory personnel within the 44th Medical Brigade, after their initial 2-week period of special training in the base laboratory in Saigon. (*Chart 14*)

Innovations

An innovation in staffing that produced outstanding results in 1968 was the assignment of an internist to the laboratory staff to head an infectious diseases department. In the 6-month period after the internist arrived, the output of diagnostic information in febrile cases more than doubled. In 1968, 29,160 diagnostic serology procedures were performed.

Veterinary laboratory officers played an important role in Vietnam. They tested ice for chlorination potability and developed serologic methods for diagnosis of melioidosis, leptospirosis, scrub typhus, and murine typhus.

The thrust of medical zoology in the laboratory system was for quality control, mainly in laboratory diagnosis of malaria and amebiasis. The malaria smears reviewed by the laboratory increased each year, from 1965 to 1969, as follows: 1965, 300; 1966, 1,199; 1967, 3,312; and 1968, 8,176. This review for quality of smear, staining, and identification of parasites was returned to each unit submitting smears, so that any deficient technique could be recognized. Where needed, special visits by central laboratory personnel were made. Similarly, materials

CHART 14—A FIELD MEDICAL LABORATORY SYSTEM IN VIETNAM

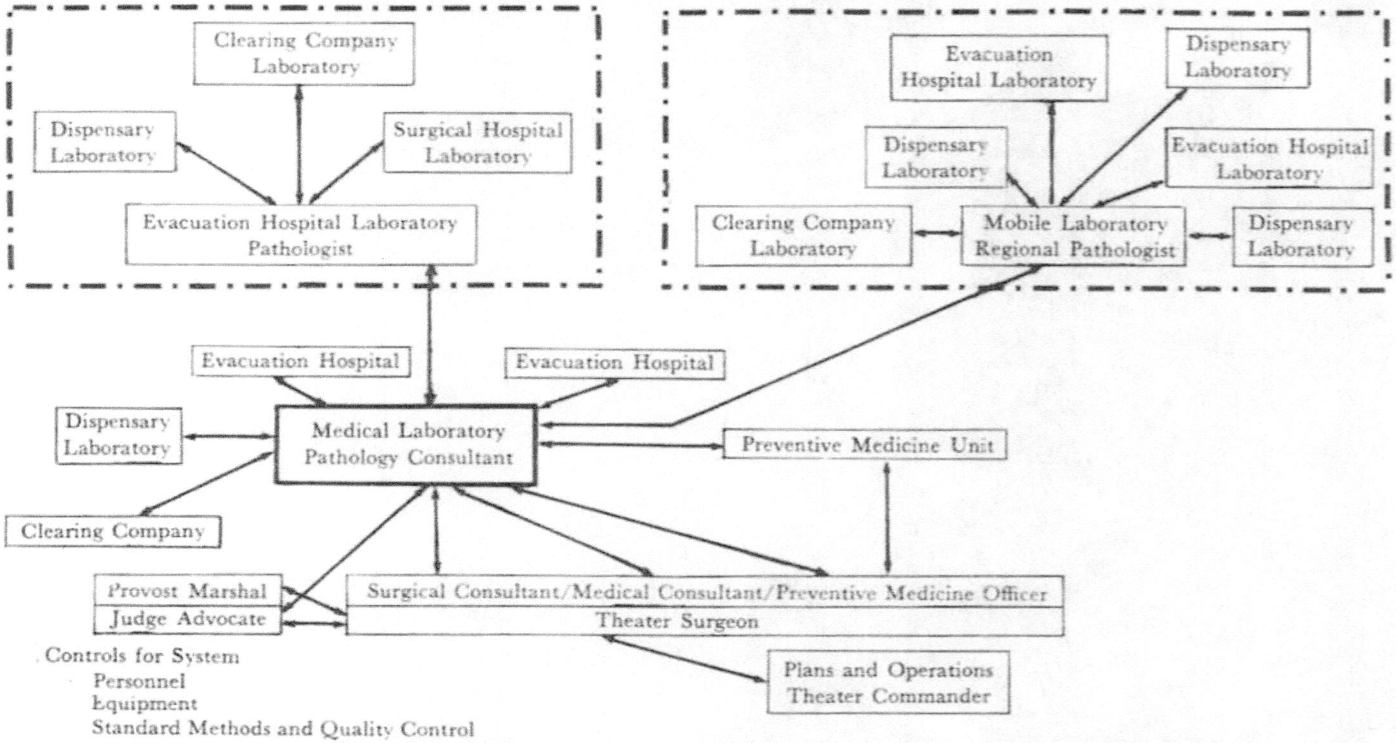

Source: H. J. Baker: Some Considerations in the Operation of a Field Medical Laboratory System. Mil. Med. 135 (5): 360, May 1970.

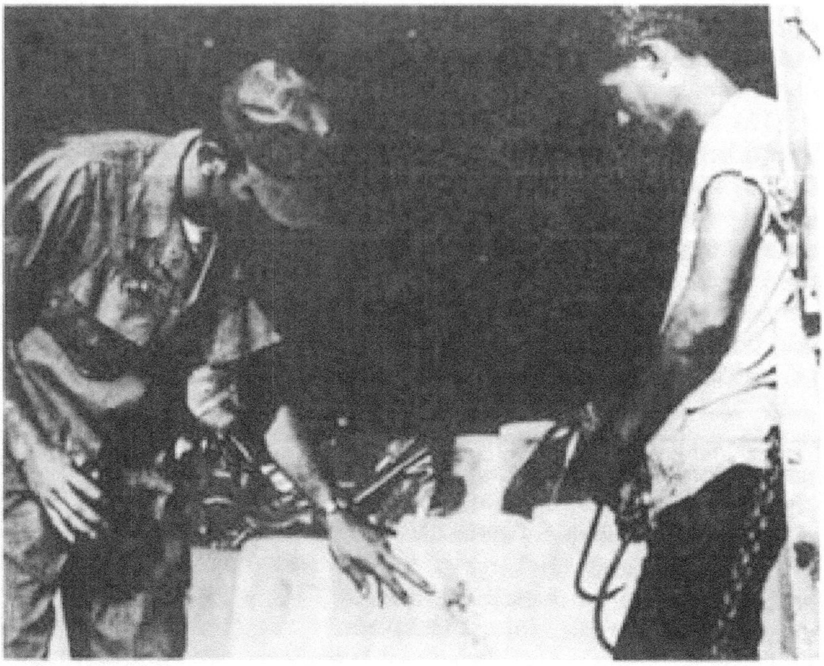

VETERINARY FOOD INSPECTOR CHECKING ICE FOR CHLORINATION AND POTABILITY, LONG BINH, VIETNAM

were provided to hospital laboratories to make trichrome stains of all stool specimens considered positive for amebic dysentery. Some specimens were submitted for review and diagnosis confirmed. The procedure for confirmation was cause for greater care on the part of technicians in field units.

Problems Surmounted

Under supervision of the base laboratory, advanced laboratory procedures were established for hospitals carrying major surgical loads where advanced intensive postoperative care was practiced. Because hospital facilities were widely scattered, with restricted land communication between them and a base laboratory and with a strictly limited number of laboratory personnel available, it was imperative that the chemistry procedures provided be essential for clinical decisions and be performed competently in forward areas.

By late 1967, surgeons recognized that advanced laboratory methodology provided information on the condition of their patients which challenged their knowledge and prior experience. Similarly, the opportunity for Army physicians to establish definitive etiological diagnoses on eight febrile diseases, being encountered for the first time in their careers, was not only a benefit to the patients but also a positive factor in professional morale.

The base laboratory maintained a courier system for specimens and reports between dispensaries, some clearing companies, all hospitals, and the 9th Medical Laboratory. Despite its imperfections, the courier system operated by virtue of the determination of the couriers. After 1968, couriers were helped in part by access to the Otter aircraft assigned to the 44th Medical Brigade.

An automatic data processing system was established to retrieve disease information by place and time. By late 1968, weekly summaries of etiological diagnostic findings in febrile disease were prepared by computer and distributed to all hospitals, preventive medicine units, and division surgeons. The summaries gave the patient's name, identification number, and unit, information which was necessary since patients often remained only a short time in facilities where the working diagnosis and treatment were initiated. Routine laboratory reports were often returned to the hospital after discharge of patients and went into their records without notice of the attending physician. The weekly summary was an attention-catching mechanism that allowed the physicians to review cases with specific findings for educational benefits on diseases occurring in Vietnam. This information served also for the purposes of disease prevention and advice for continuing military operations.

By 1968, the medical laboratory system had largely matured. It provided advanced technology where it was needed with a limited number of skilled persons strategically placed. Many persons with special skills were regularly called upon to assist in solving unusual problems. Each area pathologist was either assigned to, or closely associated with, the 9th Medical Laboratory.

The greatest need for pathologists was in supervising clinical pathology, in managing the flow of work within the laboratory, and at times even in maintaining advanced equipment. However, the most important role of the pathologist was in his relation with clinicians in understanding the nature of illness and trauma and in assuring that the most appropriate specimens reached the laboratories. A pathologist in the base laboratory was assigned the task of supervising clinical pathology throughout the 44th Medical Brigade laboratories to assure standardization of methodology.

Anatomic pathology required fewer pathologists. The greatest and most essential workload in anatomic pathology was the forensic cases. A large workload of interest to the pathologists was the surgical pathology on biopsies submitted by volunteer surgical teams working with the indigenous population. Since provision was made for frozen sections in the larger military hospitals, the processing of paraffin sections and their reading was centralized in Saigon.

The medical laboratory service in Vietnam finally reached a high level of quality service after several years. By 1970, as a result of co-ordination between the medical laboratory system and preventive medicine, a level of effectiveness comparable to that in World War II had been achieved. The primary failure had been an inordinate delay in bringing about a close co-ordination between the medical laboratory system and the preventive medicine units. Since both activities were an integral part of the laboratory system, this had not been a problem in World War II.

CHAPTER XII

Corps Services

Nursing Service

The men and women of the ANC (Army Nurse Corps) have provided nursing care of the highest quality to U.S. troops in Vietnam since mid-1962. Thirteen nurses were included on the staff of the 8th Field Hospital which arrived at Nha Trang in March 1962. Thereafter the number of nurses sent to Vietnam increased gradually as the troop buildup continued. The number reached a peak strength of 900 in January 1969, after which it fell rapidly to about 650 by July 1970 as the withdrawal of U.S. troops gained momentum.

Administration

From 1962 through 1964, when the 8th Field Hospital was the only Army hospital operating in Vietnam, the nursing service did not require the assignment of a chief nurse as a special staff adviser to the surgeon at Army component headquarters in order to function efficiently. In anticipation of the imminent buildup of Army combat and support forces, a decision was made to place a chief nurse on the staff of the USASCV surgeon early in 1965. On 3 February, Lieutenant Colonel Margaret G. Clarke, ANC, senior nurse at the 8th Field Hospital, was assigned that position as an additional duty.

Just as was true for all other Medical Department officers who wore two hats during that period, the physical separation of the 8th Field Hospital from Headquarters, USASCV, in Saigon, hindered Colonel Clarke in the accomplishment of her staff responsibilities. Consequently, when USASCV was redesignated Headquarters, USARV, on 20 July 1965, a primary duty space was authorized in the surgeon's office for a staff nurse. However, not until 15 September, when Colonel Clarke was transferred from the 8th Field Hospital to Headquarters, USARV, to assume the duties of chief nurse, was that position filled.

As chief nurse on the staff of the USARV surgeon, Colonel Clarke and her successors acted as advisers on all nursing activities, and as nursing consultants for the medical service structure in Vietnam. The scope of her responsibilities included initial assignments for incoming ANC officers and recommendations on personnel actions. That Colonel

Clarke, as the first full-time chief nurse in Vietnam, did her job well is reflected in her winning the award of "U.S. Army Nurse of the Year" in 1965.

The arrival of the 44th Medical Brigade in 1966 had no appreciable effect on the staff structure for nursing service in Vietnam. The USARV chief nurse simply assumed a second staff position as staff nurse at Headquarters, 44th Medical Brigade. By 9 March 1967, however, increases in ANC personnel and expanded nursing activities in the theater of operations warranted the assignment of a full-time nursing adviser to the staff of the commanding officer of the brigade. Consequently, Lieutenant Colonel (later Colonel) Rose V. Straley, ANC, was appointed chief nurse with responsibility for assigning and managing all ANC personnel within the brigade.

On 10 August 1967, the 44th Medical Brigade became a major subordinate command of USARV headquarters. As a result of that reorganization of the medical service structure, a position for a staff nurse in the brigade headquarters was deleted. Colonel Straley was reassigned to the 24th Evacuation Hospital with duty assignment as assistant chief nurse in the USARV surgeon's office. Once again, the USARV chief nurse donned a second hat as chief nurse of the 44th Medical Brigade.

The final reorganization of the U.S. Army medical service structure in Vietnam occurred on 1 March 1970, when Headquarters, 44th Medical Brigade, was consolidated with the USARV surgeon's office. The unified USAMEDCOMV retained a chief nurse as a staff adviser to the USARV surgeon and the USAMEDCOMV commanding general, and as nursing consultant for all U.S. Army medical facilities in Vietnam.

Assignments. The tour of duty was 1 year and this caused a problem of staff rotation in hospitals. Most hospitals arrived with a full complement of nurses whose tours ended simultaneously, necessitating complete restaffing at the end of the year. While waiting for the hospital to become operational, the original nurses were permanently assigned to units already in operation. As the hospital began to receive patients, nurses were assigned to the staff so that their eligibility for return to the United States would be staggered, thus solving the problem of mass rotation to some extent.

Assignments were often based on unit needs rather than on TOE (table of organization and equipment) authorization. Owing to rapidly changing needs, new assignments were made to a specific unit after the nurse's arrival in-country. Some factors used to meet hospital staffing requirements were the type and rapidity of admissions and dispositions, the status of enlisted staffing, and the strength or weakness of the individual officer assigned. Most nurses were assigned to hospitals and to the 6th Convalescent Center at Cam Ranh Bay. Nurses were authorized by TOE for thoracic, orthopedic, neurosurgical, maxillofacial, neuropsychiatric, renal, and other specialized teams.

The difficulty of assigning nurses was further complicated by the fact that 60 percent of the nurses assigned had less than 6 months' active duty and lacked experience in combat nursing. Vietnam became a training ground for a large number of inexperienced officers. This problem was solved by the institution of intensive training programs in each unit and continuous counseling and guidance by more experienced nurses. Army nurses also participated in professional conferences sponsored by the Allied Nations medical personnel in-country.

There was a crucial need for nurses trained in certain specialized skills. The critical need for operating-room nurses was lessened by cross training and by lending trained nurses to other hospitals in emergencies such as increases in casualties. To meet Vietnam needs, the length of the operating-room course (in the United States) was decreased from 22 to 16 weeks and offered at eight Army hospitals. The rise in the number of medical units caused by the troop buildup and high casualty rates increased the need for nurse anesthetists. Because replacements sent to Vietnam were often inexperienced, the policy of utilizing senior nurse anesthetists as instructors and traveling consultants was initiated in 1970. Ward patient care was adversely affected by the lack of field grade medical-surgical nurse supervisors; however, this shortage was alleviated by using experienced captains in supervisory positions.

Utilization of male nurses. Since 1955 men have received commissions in the Army Nurse Corps. Male nurses were assigned to organic medical units of major combat elements as well as to hospitals in Vietnam. Male nurse anesthetists were assigned to the 173d Airborne Brigade, the 101st Airborne Division, and the 1st Cavalry Division (Airmobile). They gave direct patient care, supervised nursing activities, and administered anesthesia to patients during emergency surgical procedures. One-half of all male nurses were in the clinical nursing specialties of anesthesia, operating room, and neuropsychiatry. Male nurses were used in special situations as in November 1967 when the nursing service of the 18th Surgical Hospital (MUST) was reorganized as an all-male unit in anticipation of increased enemy activity.

Combat Nursing

The highest quality of nursing care was given despite the constant threat of attack. All hospitals from the northern highlands at Pleiku to the Delta town of Vung Tau were vulnerable to enemy mortar, rocket, and small arms fire. Several, such as the 45th Surgical Hospital at Tay Ninh, the 3d Field Hospital at Saigon, and the 12th Evacuation Hospital at Cu Chi, for example, were hit one or more times. First Lieutenant

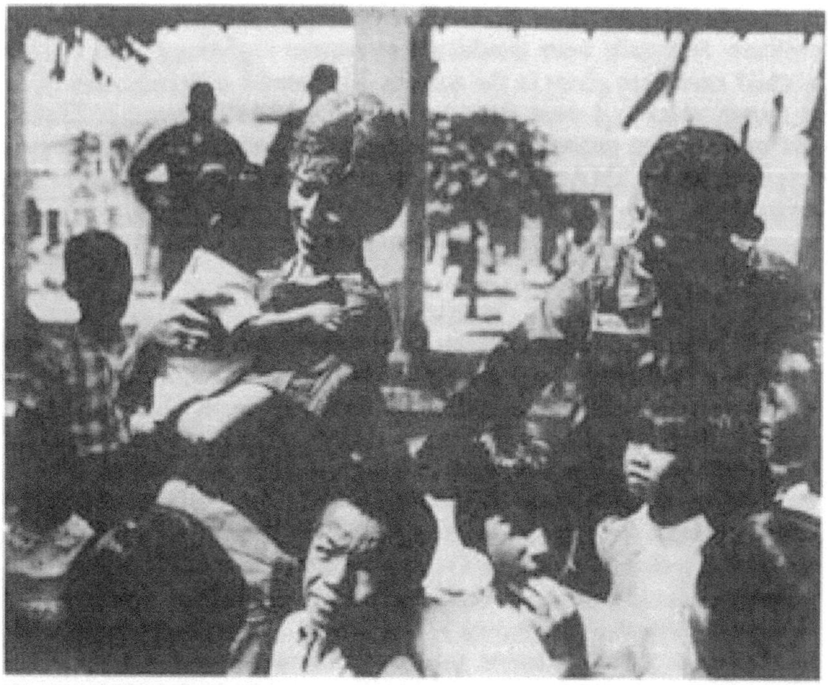

U.S. ARMY NURSES HOLD SICK CALL AT A VIETNAMESE ORPHANAGE

Sharon Anne Lane, ANC, was killed by hostile fire on 8 June 1969, while on duty at the 312th Evacuation Hospital at Chu Lai. On 11 November 1969, an intensive care ward at Fitzsimons General Hospital, Denver, Colo., was formally dedicated as the Lane Recovery Suite in memory of her service at that hospital.

The principles of good nursing remained unchanged in Vietnam but ingenuity was required to maintain high standards of nursing care. The nurses used their resourcefulness to overcome a lack of certain equipment. Stones in a Red Cross ditty bag made weights for traction, a piece of Levin's tube could be used as a drinking straw, plastic dressing wrappers served as colostomy bags, soap and intravenous bottles were used as chest drainage bottles, and items of equipment not authorized by hospital TOE were designed and constructed from scrap lumber and other materials. Improvements were constantly needed, and some were made in methods of sewage disposal and in bathing and laundry facilities. During seasonal offensives, heavier-than-normal workloads were placed on medical units, and all nurses went on 12-hour work schedules in order to maintain high standards of nursing.

Army nurses voluntarily gave medical assistance to the Vietnamese during their off-duty hours. Clinics were established and staffed by nursing personnel who gave basic care, including immunizations, to the civilians. Sick calls were conducted at various orphanages and courses in child care were given to the natives. Vietnamese nationals were hired as nurses' aides and were given intensive on-the-job training in English and basic nursing procedures. Nurses taught in Vietnamese Armed Forces hospitals, and USMACV nurses helped the Vietnamese Army train its own nurses.

Dental Service

Background

The Vietnam conflict generated new approaches for conducting warfare which extended to all phases of combat, combat support, and combat service support activities. In the latter area, changes in U.S. Army military dentistry ranged from those caused by the Vietnamese environment to others adaptable to any combat environment.

Treatment problems of the Dental Corps differ from those faced by other specialty services of the Army Medical Department, whose programs and policies are designed to cope with acute, episodic diseases and injuries. Generally, persons entering active duty are healthy young people. However, from the perspective of the Dental Corps, many of these individuals are already afflicted with chronic oral diseases. Since early in World War II, when dental standards for entry on active duty were all but eliminated, the Army has inherited from civilian life vast accumulated needs for dental care. The result was that the Army had too few dentists to remedy the results of years of neglect.

From a military perspective, the major effect of oral disease occurs when an acute, painful lesion develops. A soldier with a toothache is not a casualty in the same sense as one with a combat wound. However, if he must be absent for several days for emergency dental treatment, this absence is just as much a drain on the fighting force as is any other disability. To improve the oral health status of the military population during times of hostilities, the dental service designed programs not only to treat but also to prevent such dental emergencies.

The goal of the program during World War II and the Korean War was to treat all dental problems before the soldiers left CONUS for overseas assignments. Much of the needed treatment was accomplished, but over-all results were unsatisfactory because there were not enough dentists to perform all the necessary work, because training schedules interfered with treatment, and because new and more effective controls were needed.

In the early period of American involvement in Vietnam, dental preparation of men for duty was similar to that used in previous years. As long as the number of men involved was small, complete corrective care for all on a one-time basis was possible. But when troop strength started escalating in 1965, dental problems in preparing soldiers for combat duty also escalated. In response, new approaches were developed to support the combat missions.

Mission Concept

The major development in the concept of mission support of combat arms was the Dental Effectiveness Program. This development began after Major General Robert B. Shira, chief of the Dental Corps, visited Vietnam in the spring of 1968. He was disturbed by reports from field commanders that combat effectiveness was being disrupted by dental emergencies which incapacitated key men for as long as 7 days. General Shira's onsite evaluation resulted in the authorization of a 20-percent increase in dental officer strength to 278 officers in-country by June 1968, in the promotion of programs of mass application of preventive agents, and in the appointment of a task force to collect data on types and treatments of dental emergencies.

Preventive services, an added step in dental service activities since the Korean War, were limited because professional personnel had to perform the services. In the fall of 1968, a stannous fluoride phosphate paste, which the patient could apply himself, was developed. Semiannual applications of this paste reduced the incidence of new caries from as much as 60 percent.

The task force recommended that a dental combat effectiveness program be established at all CONUS posts conducting advanced individual training. The objectives of the program were to select individuals with critical military occupational specialties, identifying their dental needs and treating them with the least possible interference to combat training, and to develop an intermediate restorative material for fast effective sealing of deep caries.

The survey of dental emergencies disclosed an annual rate exceeding 142 per 1,000 men, which corroborated the field commanders' impressions. Since about three-fourths of the emergencies were caused by advanced caries, treatment was centered on caries likely to need attention within 12 to 18 months.

Two additional phases of dental care were started in Vietnam: in replacement centers of combat units, dental screening became part of the in-processing; and any previously overlooked dental conditions were treated immediately. In the field, dental forward area support teams provided both screening and needed dental care.

Within 9 months after the program began, the annual dental emergency rate had been reduced to 73 per 1,000 men, or by about 50 percent.

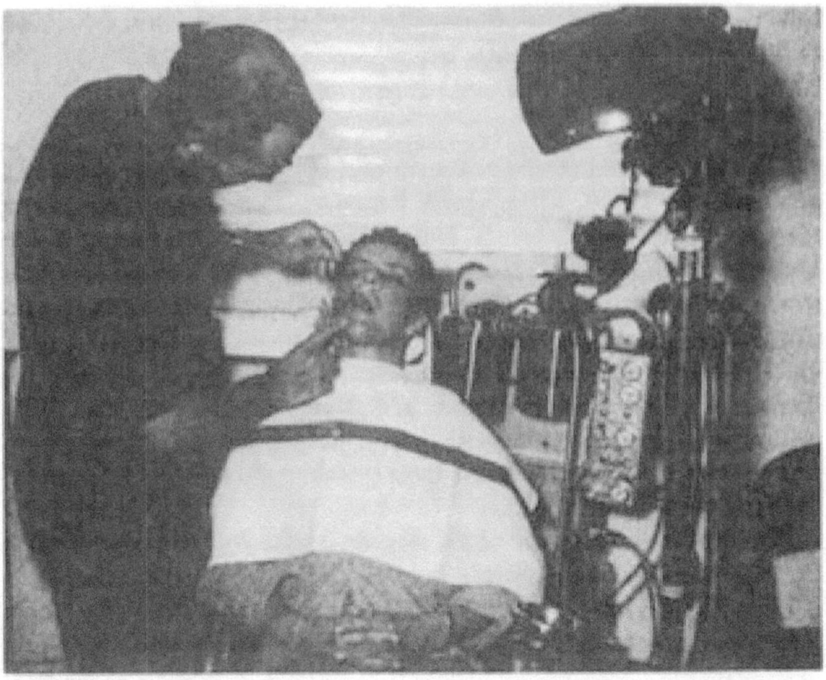

DENTAL CLINIC OF THE 85TH EVACUATION HOSPITAL IN VIETNAM

Distribution of Personnel

A new concept in the Vietnam conflict was the provision of most dental services through cellular dental units, not organic to the combat division but serving in an area support role. Team KJ, Dental Service Detachment, the first such unit, was made up of 15 dental officers, an administrative officer (Medical Service Corps), and 21 enlisted men; this team provided routine dental care. The four dental officers still assigned to the medical battalion of each division (compared to the previous 15) treated emergency conditions. Medical units, such as hospitals and dispensaries, also had organic dental officers: officers assigned to hospitals treated the hospital staff; those assigned to dispensaries treated individuals located in their immediate area.

Command and Control

At the beginning of 1965, the seven dental officers in Vietnam were assigned to the 36th Medical Detachment (KJ). Lieutenant Colonel George F. Mayer, DC, was commanding officer of the 36th; he was also dental surgeon to the 1st Logistical Command. In July 1965, the 36th was assigned officially to the 1st Logistical Command, as were other KJ teams when they arrived in-country. In December 1965, the 932d Medical Detachment (AI) assumed command over KJ teams and dental personnel organic to other medical units.

Concurrently with the arrival of the 932d in Vietnam, the position of dental surgeon was created in the Office of the Surgeon, USARV. Colonel Ralph B. Snead, DC, was assigned to this position and was also to supervise dental personnel assigned to combat divisions.

No further changes in command and control setup occurred until October 1967, when Colonel Jack P. Pollock, DC, was assigned additional duty as 44th Medical Brigade dental surgeon and technical supervisor over dental personnel in medical units as well as divisions.

Early in 1970, the USARV surgeon's office and the 44th Medical Brigade were combined to form the Medical Command, USARV. At this time, the positions previously listed as USARV dental surgeon, 44th Medical Brigade dental surgeon, and commanding officer of the 932d Medical Detachment were combined to integrate more effectively the efforts of dental personnel in KJ teams with those in nondental units.

Equipment

Among the improvements in field dental equipment were the lightweight automatic dental film processor, portable ultrasonic prophylaxis, field dental equipment set for the hygienist, more powerful air compressor, water-jet devices, and lighter and more compact field dental sets. The superior Encore portable speed dental engine was issued to more units; the power difficulties created by this engine were finally solved with the availability of additional electric power.

Dental treatment clinics were widely dispersed and ranged in size from one chair to 14 chairs; almost half of the clinics were air conditioned. They were located in tents, tropical shelters, wooden frame or concrete buildings, warehouses, quonset huts, bunkers, and mobile vans. The initial airmobile dental clinic, used by the 39th Medical Detachment (KJ) in the Pleiku area and transported by a Flying Crane helicopter, was an immediate success.

Automated records reduced the work required to maintain and gather data.

Oral Surgery

For the first time in U.S. military history, the Army Dental Corps had available both a large cadre of trained oral surgeons to provide skilled specialized surgical support, and helicopter ambulances to provide evacuation for early definitive treatment of maxillofacial injuries. New and important research contributions of the Army Institute of Dental Research to oral surgery included an improved type of surgical dressing, pulsating water-jet devices for lavage, a cold curing resin material for rapid splinting of jaw fractures, preformed silicone mandibles, and an intermediate restorative material and the ultrasonic Cavitron for peridontal disease.

Veterinary Service

The U.S. Army Veterinary Corps shares in the responsibility of safeguarding the health of the Army. In South Vietnam, during 1965–70, the Veterinary Corps performed its traditional activities under conditions which were often unlike any previously encountered by American troops. It also participated in civic action programs, and furnished advisory support to the ARVN veterinary service in an effort to improve its animal care and veterinary personnel training. Above all, however, the Veterinary Corps, in its food inspection activities and animal medicine care, met a variety of challenges and resolved difficult and complex problems posed by conditions peculiar to the Vietnamese conflict.

Food Inspection

Veterinary food inspection in Vietnam encompassed a variety of activities. The objective of these activities was to protect the health of the soldier. To achieve that objective, veterinary food inspectors carried on surveillance inspection of depot food stocks, receipt inspection of foods delivered to port facilities, and procurement inspection of indigenous ice, bread, and fresh fruits and vegetables.

Initially, all veterinary activities were carried out by the 4th Medical Detachment in Saigon. With the increase in U.S. troop strength in 1965, additional depots and ports were established throughout Vietnam, from Da Nang in the north to Vinh Long in the Delta. Only one or two food inspectors from the 4th Medical Detachment were permanently assigned to the larger of the new depots, such as that at Cam Ranh Bay, with mobile teams organized for dispatch to the smaller ones to resolve special problems. Thus, veterinary food inspection was concentrated on those major food depots which received food directly from refrigerated ships or by secondary LST shipment. Finally, in 1968, a sufficient number of veterinary food inspectors were authorized to permit total coverage for each food distribution activity.

Depot stocks. Although veterinary inspectors were primarily concerned with protecting the health of troops by preventing the consumption of unsafe foods, they were also interested in food conservation.

As more refrigerated storage facilities became available, it was possible to replace the field ration diet with one which included more dairy products as well as fresh and frozen foods. The refrigerated storage facilities available for such foods ranged from a few cold-storage warehouses remaining from French colonial days, to the self-contained, portable, walk-in boxes which became a part of each food distribution point, and to refrigerated Navy barges anchored offshore. Despite this variety, refrigerated storage was seldom of adequate capacity or temperature, and never caught up with demand. Lack of refrigerated storage frequently caused significant losses. To keep such losses to a minimum, produce on the verge of spoiling was inspected daily to determine which items to salvage and which to condemn, including items that would spoil if shipped.

Losses also occurred because depots and supply points bulged with stocks far in excess of amounts that could be consumed before deterioration. Nonperishables were stored in the open, canned goods corroded, and flour soured. With these stockpiles far greater than requirements, depot personnel were indifferent to waste. The saving factor in this subsistence supply chaos was simply the overabundance of foods which continued to flow into the country.

To bring some order out of this chaos, the 1st Logistical Command, in 1967, directed the Veterinary Corps to inspect nonperishable food stocks every 60 days. Although the Veterinary Corps favored regular, routine checks, such a workload was too great for the food inspection forces available. Surveillance inspection continued to be limited to "spot check" at irregular intervals.

Indigenous food. The purchase of indigenous foods soared after the activation of the U.S. Army Procurement Agency in May 1965. By the fall of 1966, more than $900,000 worth of produce was being purchased monthly. The amount of locally produced foods examined by veterinary inspectors rose from 50 million pounds in 1965 to 430 million in 1966. (*Table 10*) By 1967, 39 Vietnamese stores and plants had been approved as a source for the purchase of commodities, ranging from baked goods to ice.

Representatives of the Veterinary Corps and the Army Procurement Agency worked together to develop standards to govern the production of locally grown fruits and vegetables and the preparation of bread and ice. Though not as high in Vietnam as in the United States, the sanitary standards were as realistic as possible. The yardstick was: Does it endanger the health of the soldier? The manner in which the sanitary standards of the two cultures were reconciled is perhaps best illustrated in regulations governing the production of ice.

Ice was in enormous demand because of the hot, muggy climate. If ice from an approved source was not available, the soldier purchased it from the nearest Vietnamese vendor, even when it was yellow with sediment and made from water pumped from a drainage ditch. There

TABLE 10.—INSPECTION OF FOOD BY THE U.S. ARMY VETERINARY SERVICE IN VIETNAM, BY YEAR, 1965–70

Year	Grand total	Procurement inspections		Surveillance inspections	
		Passed	Rejected	Passed	Rejected [1]
	(Pounds)	*(Pounds)*	*(Pounds)*	*(Pounds)*	*(Pounds)*
1965	1, 180, 257, 008	50, 371, 193	185, 413	1, 128, 915, 986	784, 416
1966	8, 977, 251, 632	451, 415, 274	647, 125	8, 515, 523, 924	9, 665, 309
1967	13, 506, 313, 375	1, 009, 590, 408	11, 892, 306	12, 449, 488, 510	35, 342, 151
1968	10, 162, 947, 762	1, 480, 914, 582	8, 226, 612	8, 621, 357, 986	52, 448, 582
1969	7, 171, 058, 733	898, 613, 272	7, 829, 909	6, 238, 029, 734	26, 585, 818
1970 [2]	3, 667, 790, 436	549, 214, 720	1, 111, 051	3, 112, 474, 068	4, 990, 597

[1] Quantities shown represent condemnation of Government-owned foods.
[2] January–June only.
Source: Veterinary Activities Reports, 1965–70.

was evidence that contaminated ice contributed to an outbreak of viral hepatitis and that it posed a significant health hazard. To solve this problem, the Army approved purchase from Vietnamese icemaking plants which chlorinated the water to have at least 5.0 parts per million free available chlorine. Also, because attempts to sell nonpotable ice continued, all iceblocks were tested upon delivery.

Inspection of Vietnamese bakeries posed another problem. Since baking was done at night, observation during production was unsafe, even in Saigon. (Vietnamese managers claimed that Vietcong "tax collectors" chose the hours of darkness to make their rounds.) The alternative was to section samples of bread and rolls upon receipt, and examine them for insects, other extraneous matter, and "ropey dough" caused by bacterial contamination during processing of the dough. The organism involved, although nonpathogenic, caused bread to sour within 36 hours, which was often less than the time needed to distribute the bread to units. Contaminated bakeries were suspended until cleanup procedures had eliminated the problem and the bread kept for 96 hours at ambient temperatures.

Perishable food at resupply points. No single factor so profoundly affected the fresh food supply and distribution procedures as did the Sea-Land van deliveries that began in December 1967. These vans, loaded at west coast ports on ships modified for them, were self-contained refrigerators which could maintain optimum temperatures for the items transported. Wheels, bolted in place upon arrival, made the vans mobile. Van refrigeration units operated on bottled gas, or from an outside source of electric power. The advantages of the vans were obvious: better temperature control, less handling of product, and faster loading and off-loading, with issue made directly from vans to ration trucks. This revolutionary procedure made possible volume delivery of such highly perishable items as lettuce, pears, tomatoes, and melons.

Food inspectors made daily checks of the vans parked in Sea-Land yards, recording temperatures and noting product condition. This information, supplied to the 1st Logistical Command, permitted immediate response and centralized control of perishable items. In addition, veterinary out-turn reports forwarded directly to CONUS provided procuring activities with feedback data. As road security improved, vans made direct delivery to the supply points of all but the more remote combat units.

With increased utilization of Sea-Land vans and the advent of palletized shipping containers, the veterinary food inspection specialists authorized for Transportation Terminal Commands in Vietnam could not be fully utilized at the ports, for to dismantle palletized and weatherproofed packaged items at dockside would compromise the protection

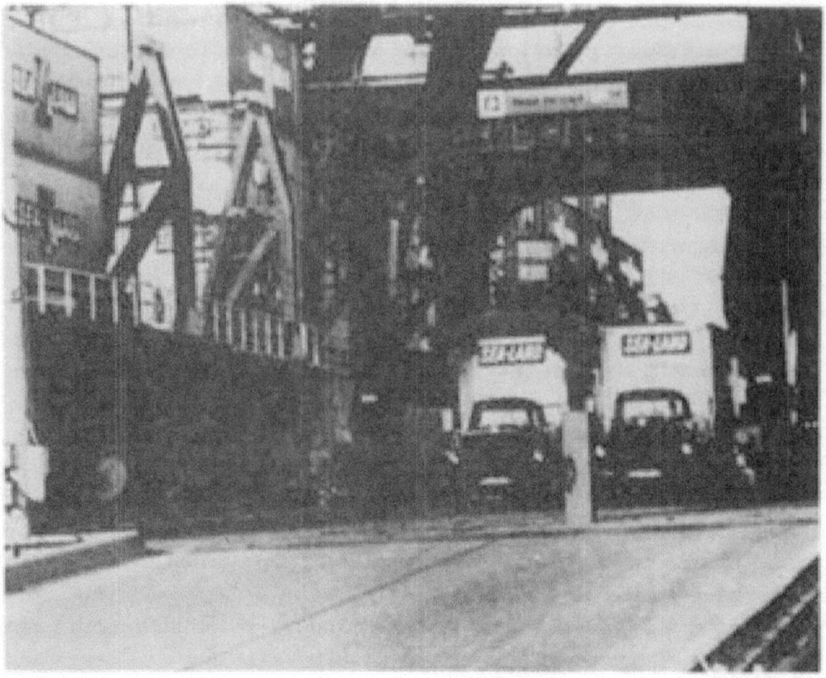

PACECO PORTAINER GANTRY CRANES *unload refrigerated vans onto 10-ton trucks from the deck of a freighter, Cam Ranh Bay, Vietnam.*

provided against the elements and against pilferage. Furthermore, because port operations were either "feast or famine," food inspection resources could be better utilized in nearby depots. Accordingly, an informal agreement was made with Transportation Terminal commanders, making food inspection personnel organic to these commands available to the major veterinary food inspection unit in that area. This move materially aided the over-all inspection effort.

Animal Medicine

Routine care. Initially, in 1965, routine professional veterinary care for military dogs in Vietnam was provided by three small veterinary food inspection detachments then in-country. Each of these units was authorized one veterinary animal specialist, in addition to its food inspection specialists. At that time, approximately 350 Army and Marine Corps sentry dogs were assigned to some 10 locations throughout the country.

With the buildup of U.S. forces and the accompanying increased use of dogs in field operations, the dog population rose from the 350 in 1965, to more than 1,200 in 1968, dispersed widely throughout Vietnam.

With more veterinary support required in the forward areas, additional veterinary detachments arrived in Vietnam, but without a comparable increase in the numbers of animal specialists. Veterinary food inspectors from the forward detachments were used to augment the small number of these specialists. Utilizing the services of these additional veterinary enlisted men was, at first, hampered by their inexperience in animal medicine and by the lack of veterinary medical equipment sets in the food inspection units. This situation was remedied by training food inspectors locally in certain animal specialist skills, and by obtaining equipment from the veterinary hospital and dispensary detachments.

The need for fewer food inspectors and for more animal specialists and animal medical equipment sets in Vietnam constituted a significant change in the operation of veterinary service detachments. To reflect this need, appropriate changes were subsequently made in the veterinary service tables of organization and equipment.

Hospitalization and evacuation. The 4th Medical Detachment maintained a small-animal clinic in Saigon for the emergency care and treatment of military dogs and for mascots and animals privately owned by U.S. Army troops and other authorized personnel. All animals requiring extensive treatment were evacuated to Saigon, except Marine Corps dogs which were evacuated to Da Nang.

In January 1966, the 936th Veterinary Detachment (ID), a veterinary small-animal hospital, arrived at the Tan Son Nhut Airbase to provide definitive medical care and hospitalization for all military dogs in the II, III, and IV CTZ. Additionally, it provided a consultation service to the field, monitoring all dog medical records, requisitioning and issuing all veterinary drugs to area veterinarians, and collecting and evaluating veterinary military dog statistics. On 19 October 1966, a small-animal dispensary detachment, the 504th Medical Detachment (IE), arrived in Da Nang. Although organized as a dispensary, this unit provided complete veterinary service for scout and sentry dogs in the entire I CTZ. In 1966, also, the veterinary department of the 9th Medical Laboratory became operational, making available comprehensive veterinary laboratory diagnostic services and investigations of animal diseases of military and economic interest.

In 1968, with the arrival of additional small-animal dispensary detachments, the three echelons of veterinary care and treatment of military dogs—unit, dispensary, and hospital—became clearly established. Particular emphasis was placed on improving administrative procedures to provide more definitive data on the health of military dogs. An expanded monthly morbidity and mortality reporting system was developed, and completion of detailed admission reports for hospitalized dogs was stressed.

Deployment of scout dogs in 1966 resulted in casualties suffered in action. To insure prompt treatment, dogs were evacuated by air to the 936th Veterinary Detachment (ID). Handlers were evacuated with their dogs, and remained with them until treatment was completed.

During 1969, difficulties were encountered in evacuating military dogs from dog units and veterinary dispensaries to veterinary hospital facilities. Accordingly, a firm evacuation policy was established. All dogs requiring treatment for more than 7 days were evacuated. In addition, a veterinary medical regulator was designated to direct the flow of dogs to the hospital facilities. Evacuation of military dogs was co-ordinated with the Air Force and with medical units utilizing ground and air ambulances.

In 1969, also, the high incidence and prolonged course of Tropical Canine Pancytopenia left some military dog units unable to perform adequately. The remedy was establishment of dog-holding detachments at the two veterinary hospitals. Dogs to be hospitalized for 15 days or longer were transferred to the dog-holding detachment, thereby enabling the dog unit to requisition replacement dogs.

Medical problems. Canine disabilities most frequently seen, in addition to wounds from hostile action, were heat exhaustion, ectoparasites and endoparasites, myiasis, nasal leeches, and dermatoses of varying etiology. Heartworms posed a potentially severe canine disease problem. Cases of microfilaria were as high as 40 percent in some scout dog platoons, although few animals exhibited clinical signs of disease. The incidence of hookworms was comparable to that of heartworms, and was frequently manifested by clinical signs. Outbreaks of disease resembling leptospirosis occurred; one incident involved 55 dogs, but laboratory examinations did not confirm the clinical diagnosis. Ticks, a persistent problem throughout Vietnam, required equally persistent control measures.

Tropical Canine Pancytopenia, an unusual disease characterized by hemorrhage, severe emaciation, pancytopenia, and high mortality, broke out in 1968, in U.S. military dogs in Vietnam. Know first as IHS (Idiopathic Hemorrhagic Syndrome) and ultimately as TCP (Tropical Canine Pancytopenia), the disease seriously jeopardized the operational efficiency of combat units dependent on military dogs. Between July 1968 and December 1970, about 220 U.S. military dogs, primarily German Shepherds, died of the disease, and it was the contributing reason for the euthanasia of many others. Near the end of 1969, a program of tetracycline and supportive therapy for 14 days, based on recommendations from the WRAIR laboratories in Saigon, was initiated for all TCP cases. This therapy returned to duty approximately 50 percent of the dogs treated for the disease.

Beginning in May 1969, "red tongue," a nonfatal, nonsuppurative glossitis, occurred in a significant number of military dogs. The glossitis was often accompanied by excessive salivation, gingivitis and edema of the gums, and, at times, a serious conjunctivitis. The condition is extremely painful, and affected dogs could eat and drink only with difficulty. In most instances, the signs regressed and the dogs returned to normal in 3 to 7 days. The etiology of the condition has not been established.

Acute glossitis in scout dogs spread throughout Vietnam during 1970. Morbidity rates as high as 100 percent in some platoons made these units noneffective for periods up to 2 weeks.

Up to 1966, the Army veterinary rabies control program was primarily restricted to vaccination of military dogs, pets, and mascots. In August of that year a co-ordinated rabies program was put in operation. Vaccination clinics were held, often as far forward as medical clearing stations. Three major difficulties were recognized: the enormous number of pets acquired by Americans, the large number of small units throughout the country, and the absence of meaningful civilian rabies control programs.

In September 1967, standard procedures were established for the control of pets and the program was widely publicized by radio and television, stressing the dangers of rabies. More than 7,000 animal vaccinations were reported for 1967, the majority being rabies immunizations. Nevertheless, in that year only half of the animals owned by U.S. soldiers were vaccinated. The significant problem here was that many men were located in small detachments scattered among the Vietnamese communities, where pet control was essentially nonexistent. One countermeasure was to vaccinate Vietnamese dogs around U.S. military installations, thereby lessening the chance of dogs on these bases coming into contact with rabid animals. Where possible, dogs were vaccinated on Vietnamese military installations. Also, with the requirement that soldiers pay for having their pets vaccinated, many were reluctant to immunize or identify their animals.

The Vietnam experience showed the need for free rabies vaccinations for animals privately owned by U.S. personnel, to assure an unhampered, comprehensive disease control program. Toward this end, with the existing active combat conditions in Vietnam, the Army waived the provisions of the regulation which required payment to the Government for immunization and quarantine of such privately owned animals.

Army Medical Specialist Corps Services

Three AMSC (Army Medical Specialist Corps) officers (two dietitians and one physical therapist) were assigned to Vietnam in the spring of 1966. There was no authorization for these officers in existing TOE's (tables of organization and equipment) for field and evacuation hospitals, but because hospitals in Vietnam operated as fixed installations, providing essentially the same services as station and general hospitals in the continental United States, the need for dietitians and physical therapists was recognized. The relatively short periods for which patients were hospitalized in Vietnam precluded the long-range rehabilitation programs provided by occupational therapists; however, occupational therapy was used extensively in caring for patients evacuated to Japan. During the buildup of medical support in Vietnam in fiscal year 1966, 30 AMSC officers—13 dietitians, 10 physical therapists, and seven occupational therapists—were assigned to hospitals in Japan.

The two dietitians assigned to Vietnam in 1966 acted as consultants to hospitals in establishing food service programs. Major (later Lieutenant Colonel) Patricia Accountius, dietitian, was originally assigned to the 3d Field Hospital in Saigon, but was soon given the additional post of dietary consultant for the 44th Medical Brigade, 1st Logistical Command. Captain James Stuhmuller was assigned at the medical group level. Major (later Lieutenant Colonel) Barbara Gray, physical therapist, was assigned to the 17th Field Hospital, Saigon, but also acted as consultant to hospitals throughout the command. Because of the contributions made by these officers to the improvement of hospital food service and to the in-country rehabilitation of patients, requests were received for the assignment of additional AMSC personnel.

In the spring of 1967, four dietitians and 10 physical therapists were assigned. The senior dietitian continued to act as dietary consultant to the 44th Medical Brigade and dietitians were assigned to headquarters staff of medical groups. Physical therapists were utilized in evacuation and field hospitals, with the senior therapist having the additional duty as consultant at the brigade level.

The utilization of physical therapists remained essentially unchanged. In August 1967, the dietary staff adviser of the 44th Medical Brigade was given the additional duty as consultant to the USARV surgeon. With the formation of USAMEDCOMV (Provisional) in March 1970, the dietary staff adviser was assigned to the office of the USARV surgeon. Another major organizational change affecting dietitians occurred in July 1968, when food service sections were made separate elements within each medical group headquarters. Staff dietitians, designated as primary staff officers, food service warrant officers (food advisers) and hospital food service noncommissioned officers (food service supervisors) constituted the section staffs. Concurrent transfer of all food service functions and personnel from the S-4 Section to the newly created food service section increased the effectiveness of dietitians as consultants at the group level. The maximum authorization for AMSC officers in Vietnam was 17, which included 12 physical therapists and five dietitians. The largest number of AMSC officers serving in Vietnam at any given time was 21.

Dietitians

Because a shortage of dietitians precluded their assignment at the hospital level, the concept of the group or "shared" dietitian provided the best utilization of these specialists. Dietetic supervision of several hospitals was easily accomplished because of the proximity of hospitals within each group and the availability of air travel. The use of the Army Master Cycle Menu (Field Ration Menu) in all medical facilities, coupled with the necessity for centralizing food requirements for modified diet food items to assure logistical support, lent itself to the concept of centralized planning and control.

A major accomplishment of dietitians in Vietnam was in menu planning and the procurement of adequate subsistence supplies for hospitals. At the request of the 1st Logistical Command and in co-operation with the Defense Supply Agency, the 44th Medical Brigade dietitian, in 1966 developed a 28-day cycle master menu which was used by both field and hospital messes in Vietnam. A hospital master menu was also developed which provided meal plans for the approximately 14 types of modified diets commonly served in hospitals. These menus were updated as a wider variety of food and equipment became available. With the excellent support of the subsistence section of the 1st Logistical Command, early problems in availability of subsistence items were largely resolved, and hospitals were given first priority for food issues when shortages did occur.

Staff dietitians reviewed, analyzed, and evaluated space design and layouts to upgrade medical food service facilities. By personal visits to various supply depots, they were able to locate and arrange for delivery of garrison-type mess equipment to hospital messes. By the end of 1968, TOE food service equipment in all hospitals within the 44th Medical Brigade, with the exception of the I Corps Tactical Zone, had been replaced by garrison-type equipment.

Improvements in assigning, utilizing, and training enlisted men and civilians resulted in high-quality food service to hospitalized patients. Originally, hospital tables of organization and equipment did not authorize hospital food service enlisted personnel (MOS 94F40 and 94B30), and as a result, many military cooks and mess stewards assigned to hospitals were without previous experience in this specialized type of feeding. Many food service warrant officers (MOS 941A), who were directly in charge of food service at individual medical facilities, also lacked experience in this type of food service. Conversely, hospital-trained food service personnel were often assigned to troop-feeding facilities. Through personal screening of food service personnel arriving in-country, this situation was partially alleviated, and in 1967, modified tables of organization and equipment reflected the need for hospital-trained enlisted men in food service sections. The accomplishments of many of these men in upgrading the quality of food service to patients deserve special recognition.

Food service to bed patients remained a problem. Electric carts used to deliver bulk food to the wards were not suitable for use in hospitals which did not have covered ramps and cement walkways. Many hospitals continued to use insulated containers to hand-carry food to ward areas. There was no provision in tables of organization and equipment for ward tray service attendants, and overtaxed nursing staffs often had the responsibility for assembling trays on wards and delivering food to patients. In 1969, authorization was received to employ Vietnamese for this purpose.

Dietitians provided assistance to Allied personnel serving in Vietnam. The USARV dietary consultant, working with the 1st Logistical Command II Field Force food service consultant and the G-4 of the Royal Thai Army Volunteer Forces, developed a more acceptable ration for the Thai Army and assisted in training programs for Thai food service personnel. At the request of the U.S. Army Engineer Command, Vietnam, dietitians assisted Free World forces from Korea and Australia with their cantonment mess programs in procuring equipment and in training personnel in the use of the equipment in food preparation.

Physical Therapists

The work performed by the first physical therapist assigned to Vietnam in 1966 demonstrated the value of this type of treatment for certain injuries, particularly soft-tissue injuries to extremities. The need for additional physical therapists was evident from the many requests for their services from physicians throughout the country. After evaluation of the numbers and types of patients who could benefit from physical therapy in USARV medical facilities, the decision was made in 1967 to assign physical therapists to field and evacuation hospitals and to the 6th Convalescent Center. The senior therapist, in her capacity as Brigade consultant, had the responsibility for constantly assessing facilities and workloads and for assigning incoming officers and enlisted men to hospitals most in need of their services.

Malassignments often occurred with physical therapy specialists (MOS 91J20). Since no authorizations existed, trained specialists arriving in-country were often assigned in their secondary military occupational specialty. Until this deficiency was corrected, records of incoming personnel were carefully screened and qualified individuals were diverted to medical facilities where their specialized training and experience could be better utilized.

The primary treatment goal of physical therapy was the rehabilitation of patients who were capable of being returned to duty. For patients requiring evacuation, treatment was aimed toward starting basic rehabilitation procedures which could be continued throughout the evacuation process. Because of the relatively short periods of hospitalization of patients in Vietnam, physical therapy during the initial years was largely limited to ward-treatment programs, although a number of outpatients were treated in some hospitals. Because commanding officers were so pleased to have the services of physical therapists, they were most co-operative in providing space for clinics and helping to procure equipment. As facilities and equipment were improved, the types of treatment available in physical therapy clinics were also expanded. More long-term treatment programs, particularly for Vietnamese patients, were initiated, and a great deal of emphasis was placed on training Vietnamese technicians in physical therapy techniques and procedures. Physical therapists volunteered their services to civilian hospitals and rehabilitation centers to assist in treatment of civilian casualties. In May 1970, at the request of the U.S. Military Assistance Command, Vietnam, a physical therapist was assigned to that command to participate in rehabilitation programs being established in ARVN hospitals. Her primary responsibility was training Vietnamese to conduct these programs.

CHAPTER XIII

Medical Assistance to Vietnamese Civilians

U.S. civilian medical aid programs began in the early years of support in Vietnam. As the U.S. military commitment grew throughout the 1960's, new and expanded programs were developed. Through such efforts as PHAP (Provincial Health Assistance Program), MILPHAP (Military Provincial Health Assistance Program), MEDCAP (Medical Civic Action Program), and CWCP (Civilian War Casualty Program), medical aid in increasing amounts and effectiveness was given to the people of Vietnam.

Provincial Health Assistance Program

The Agency for International Development initiated a program in the early 1960's to supplement the health services of the Vietnamese. A major objective of PHAP was to improve the training of Vietnamese physicians, nurses, and medical technicians. Others were to expand and improve Vietnamese hospitals and dispensaries and to eradicate malaria.

Under the auspices of AID, surgical teams of U.S. civilian physicians, nurses, and technicians were sent to Vietnamese provincial hospitals. The first of these teams arrived at the provincial hospital in Can Tho in the summer of 1962; shortly thereafter, teams were assigned to the hospitals at Nha Trang and Da Nang. Surgical units, consisting of two operating rooms, a central supply area, and a four-bed recovery ward, were constructed adjacent to the provincial hospital where the team was assigned.

Despite the valiant efforts of the U.S. teams, augmented by those from New Zealand, South Korea, the Philippines, and other nations of the Free World, the broad and ambitious aims of PHAP could not be realized. The task of substantially improving health care in an underdeveloped nation was difficult enough. Compounded by civil strife and guerrilla warfare, it became impossible.

Military Provincial Health Assistance Program

The increase in military medical resources which accompanied the buildup of U.S. combat troops in 1965 permitted an expansion of the effort to improve the health of Vietnamese civilians. In conjunction

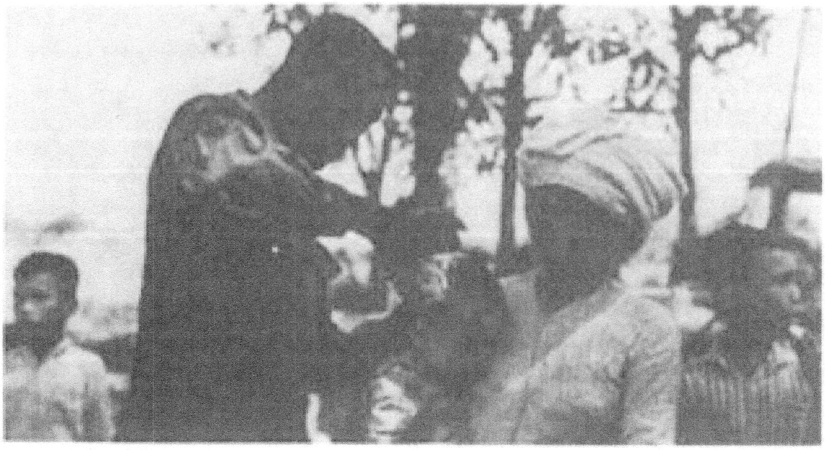

A MEDCAP Mission in Vietnam

with the buildup, the Secretary of Defense directed the services to prepare a program to aid the civilian health effort in Vietnam. The new program, which initially employed Army military medical teams in direct aid to civilians, was MILPHAP. It was developed jointly by AID and USMACV.

The first MILPHAP teams went into operation in Vietnam in November 1965. Each team was composed of three physicians, one medical administrative officer, and 12 enlisted technicians. A MILPHAP team was assigned to a Vietnamese provincial hospital where its work was under the supervision of the provincial chief of medicine. By early 1966, six teams were functioning in provincial centers and the decision was made to add 15 teams to the program. The number increased to eight Army, seven Navy, and seven Air Force MILPHAP teams by May 1968. At the end of 1970, teams were assigned to 25 of the 44 provinces.

Sent to both provincial hospitals and district dispensaries, the units provided continuity in medical care at permanent civilian medical facilities. By augmenting or, in some cases, replacing the Vietnamese medical staff, MILPHAP teams assisted in clinical, medical, and surgical care. They provided a permanent source of support for local public health programs. With the co-operation of the chiefs of medicine in the provinces, the teams established a program of evacuation for patients to those Vietnamese and American medical installations which had a greater capacity for extended treatment.

The MILPHAP teams were reorganized in 1969 to make them more responsive to the requirements of the varying sizes of the medical installations to which they are assigned. The reorganization provided more surgeons and nurses with levels of skill appropriate to the medical facility in which they served. By the end of 1970, the program supported a total of 30 Vietnamese Ministry of Health hospitals, in addition to its work in district and smaller Vietnamese medical installations.

A major objective of MILPHAP was to improve the medical skills of the Vietnamese. In 1970 alone, for example, more than 700 Vietnamese nurses received training in hospitals supported by MILPHAP teams. Through this type of training, the program advanced toward its primary goal, the development of an independent, self-sustaining health service program in Vietnam.

A medical policy co-ordinating committee was established in 1965 to plan and co-ordinate the growing number of medical programs involving aid to Vietnamese civilians. Headed jointly by the Assistant Director for Public Health, AID, and by the Surgeon, USMACV, the committee also included the surgeons of the USMACV component commands. Efforts to eliminate duplication in the administration of civilian health programs between AID and USMACV resulted in the establishment of joint USMACV–AID working committees in 1968. The committees formulated joint plans for hospital construction, medical supply, medical education and training, preventive medicine, and public health. By including military and civilian Vietnamese medical officials as members of the committees, policy makers laid a basis for the future assumption of responsibility for these programs by the Vietnamese themselves.

Medical Civic Action Program

The best known of the various programs in Vietnam for medical civil assistance was MEDCAP. Developed from a joint proposal by the American Embassy, Saigon, and USMACV made in 1962, MEDCAP began operation under the auspices of the Department of the Army in January 1963.

The primary objective of MEDCAP was to provide increased outpatient care for Vietnamese civilians living in rural areas. American and Vietnamese military medical personnel were used in the program, a major goal of which was to increase mutual respect and co-operation between the military forces and the civilian population.

Originally, medical assistance was provided by U.S. military advisory teams and Special Forces personnel; as the program grew, regular American military units participated. Initial MEDCAP organization comprised some 127 U.S. Army medical personnel, working in three teams. Later, medical personnel came from all the U.S. military services in Vietnam, although the Army continued to administer the program and support it logistically.

Although some improvisation was necessary due to local needs and conditions, the MEDCAP teams normally traveled to hamlets and villages with their ARVN counterparts and established temporary health stations, of dispensary size, to provide medical care for the inhabitants. Through the operation of these teams, Vietnamese medical personnel were also trained in medical techniques.

In contrast to MILPHAP, the MEDCAP team was a mobile unit which visited a village for a short period of time, treating civilians only on an outpatient basis. Although each team was supervised by a medical officer, the enlisted medical personnel provided most of the direct effort. MEDCAP can properly be regarded as complementing the more permanent operation of the MILPHAP team. While the latter might operate a surgical facility in a provincial hospital, or assist in the renovation of local medical facilities, the former team worked on a "one-day visit" basis in areas where more permanent medical aid was impractical.

The buildup of U.S. forces in Vietnam beginning in 1965 afforded the opportunity both to expand and to extend MEDCAP. Direct participation in the program by American and Free World military units of battalion size and larger became known as MEDCAP II; the original program which continued was then called MEDCAP I. Even in the expanded effort, however, U.S. personnel were directed, unless it was impractical, to conduct their medical civic action effort through a member of the RVNAF medical service or the Vietnamese civilian government medical authorities. MEDCAP retained the objective of eventually enabling the Vietnamese to assume the complete burden of medical care for their own people.

To support the expanded effort, a new supply system was developed for MEDCAP in July 1967. Previously, medical supplies had been furnished through the RVNAF medical depot system, but difficulties of distance and co-ordination made this means of supply increasingly unwieldy. Under new procedures, MEDCAP units were authorized to requisition material directly through the regular U.S. Army supply channels. Supply levels were also increased in recognition of the larger number of MEDCAP projects.

The extent of the MEDCAP program in Vietnam was remarkable. Both American and Free World forces participated in it, often on a volunteer basis. On many occasions, U.S. medical personnel devoted their free time to MEDCAP activities. In the later years of the program, when time and circumstances allowed, more extensive treatment than outpatient care was given. From 1 December 1967 to 31 March 1968, a monthly average of 188,441 civilians received outpatient treatment from personnel of the program. A monthly average of 17,686 Vietnamese were immunized in the same period. By 1970, the MEDCAP II program alone treated an average of 150,000 to 225,000 outpatients per month.

Both U.S. dental and veterinary military personnel participated in the MEDCAP program with equally gratifying results. The dental contribution to the program is often termed "DENTCAP." An attempt to alleviate the dental defects of the Vietnamese people was made by dental officers and enlisted technicians. During the 1967–68 period previously mentioned, dental treatments under the program averaged approximately 15,000 per month.

In a country as predominantly rural and agricultural as Vietnam, veterinary activities were of great importance in any medical civic action program. U.S. Army veterinary personnel provided much aid in swine husbandry and animal disease control as early as 1966. Sometimes called VETCAP, veterinary participation in MEDCAP increased in the following years. Treatment of sick and wounded animals, cattle vaccination, and guidance in the care and feeding of swine and cattle were all part of VETCAP activities. A rabies control project was also undertaken. During 1967 alone, a total of 21,391 animals in civilian communities were immunized against rabies, and 2,254 farm animals were treated for various diseases.

Civilian War Casualty Program

The success of MILPHAP and MEDCAP only partially met the medical needs of the Vietnamese people. As the tempo of the war increased in 1967, the growing problem of civilian war casualties called for new efforts. Estimates of 50,000 such casualties a year indicated that existing Vietnamese medical resources would be overwhelmed in providing care for these victims.

After some discussion U.S. Government officials assigned to the Department of Defense the mission of providing additional care for Vietnamese civilian casualties. The U.S. Army was directed to begin a program to this end, and in April 1967, a detailed plan drawn up by USMACV was approved by the Secretary of Defense. The CWCP was provided with the resources necessary to construct additional hospitals in Vietnam to care for civilian casualties.

A temporary allocation of 300 beds in U.S. Army hospitals in Vietnam was made, with this number increased to 400 in December 1967. Three Army hospitals, the 27th Surgical at Chu Lai, the 95th Evacuation at Da Nang, and the 29th Evacuation at Can Tho, with a total bed capacity of 1,100, were then designated as CWCP hospitals. American military medical personnel were assigned to the program, and plans were made for additional hospital construction.

The original intent of CWCP was that medical installations assigned to the program would remain separate from the U.S. military hospital system in Vietnam. Because of the reluctance of Vietnamese civilians to leave their home areas for treatment in distant hospitals, and because of the increase in civilian casualties during the Tet Offensive in early 1968, the program was modified. Treatment of Vietnamese civilians in U.S.

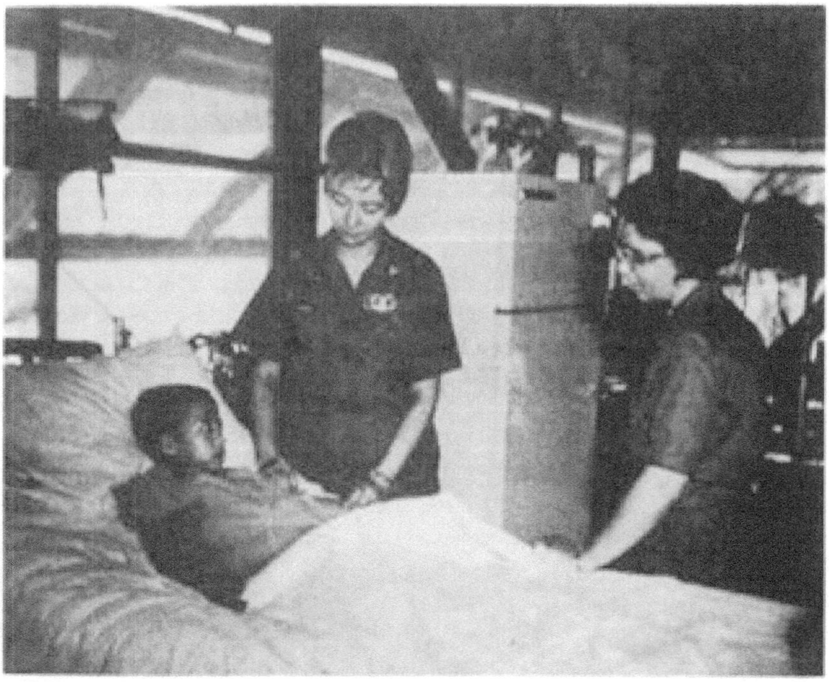

A VIETNAMESE CIVILIAN UNDERGOING TREATMENT AT A U.S. ARMY HOSPITAL IN VIETNAM

military hospitals had been authorized on a limited basis since the buildup of American forces and installations in the country. During the period of the Tet hostilities, a civilian patient load higher than normal was assumed by all U.S. military hospitals. This system of "joint occupancy" by American military and Vietnamese civilian patients was found to be the more practical alternative to a separate CWCP hospital system.

Under this system, Vietnamese civilians more readily accepted extended treatment at a location near their home areas. Additionally, administrative and evacuation procedures were simplified under the system and construction requirements were lessened. Acting on the direction of the Secretary of Defense, USMACV incorporated the previously designated CWCP hospitals into the U.S. military hospital system in April 1968. Vietnamese civilian patients were authorized treatment at all military hospitals on a space available basis. As the number of American forces was reduced during 1970, a requirement to maintain 600 beds in U.S. Army hospitals for CWCP was established. Provisions for periodic re-evaluation of the facilities needed for the program were included in this requirement.

In late 1968, USMACV and AID jointly proposed that Vietnamese military and civilian hospitals be merged. The proposal called for the merger of RVNAF sector hospitals with the civilian provincial hospitals in areas where the move would improve medical service. In a three-stage implementation of the plan following its adoption, 13 hospitals were chosen for immediate merger, 12 more needing minor reorganization and rehabilitation were added thereafter, and certain Vietnamese Government buildings were converted to hospital use. The entire program integrated the hospital systems in 26 of the 44 provinces. The consolidation enabled the Vietnamese people and their armed forces to receive the maximum care available from their medical resources.

CHAPTER XIV

Summary and Conclusions

The thirteen preceding chapters in this monograph present a review of the major areas of Medical Department activity in support of the U.S. Army in Vietnam, as derived from a variety of official documents. This final chapter, on the other hand, includes value judgments related to these activities, their successes and weaknesses, and highlights some of the more significant lessons learned. These opinions are based upon extensive review of official records and reports as well as on my own experience and observations during two tours of duty as a senior medical officer in Vietnam, interspersed with two tours of duty in the Office of The Surgeon General.

Medical Command and Control System

The preferred organization for employing and controlling military medical resources is the vertical medical command and control system which reached its epitome in Vietnam. Medical service is an integrated system with its treatment, evacuation, hospitalization, supply, service, and communications components. It is not a subsystem of logistics, nor is it a subsystem of personnel.

To achieve maximum effectiveness and efficiency in medical service support, with the utmost economy in the utilization of scarce health care resources, there must be strong professional medical control from the most forward to the most rearward echelon. The commander of the medical command, regardless of echelon, should function as the staff surgeon to the responsible supported commander. Medical capability must not be fragmented among subordinate elements but rather centrally directed and controlled by the senior medical commander. No nonmedical commanders should be interposed between the medical commander and the line commander actually responsible for the health of the command. Specifically, logistical commanders, with their broad materiel-related functions, should not be made responsible for a task so critical and so uniquely professional as the provision of health services. The well-being and care of the individual soldier must not be submerged in, or subordinated to, the system responsible for the supply and maintenance of his equipment. The issues involved are too great to risk failure or marginal accomplishment.

Health of the Command

The health of the U.S. Army in Vietnam has been excellent. A major consideration in the decision to commit U.S. forces in Southeast Asia was the concern that disease in that area would decimate our troops, and that active combat operations would be impossible. This was not the case. A major contributing factor to the well-being of U.S. troops was the recognition that a 6-week period of adjustment and acclimatization was needed. This "precommitment" period provided, most definitely, one of the lessons learned in Vietnam.

Empirically, it has been observed that it takes about 5 days to adjust to the significant time zone changes and to develop a new diurnal cycle. It also takes 2 to 3 weeks to acclimatize to the heat and humidity of the Tropics, if troop stresses are gradually increased. A total of approximately 6 weeks is required to develop a "relative biological acclimatization" to the types of infectious organisms encountered in the new environment. This 6-week period of adjustment and acclimatization was a necessity; command recognized it as a physiological and biological reality, and senior commanders in Vietnam postponed commitment to major combat operations accordingly.

During this 6-week period, troops spent their time profitably. They learned again to live in the field, mess personnel became more efficient in field sanitation, and all the new arrivals developed a keen awareness of the problem of health and a greater appreciation of the necessity for a vigorous preventive medicine program—both by command and by the individual.

The diseases encountered in Vietnam were those which have plagued all armies through the years: fever of undetermined origin, diarrhea, upper respiratory infections, dermatological conditions, and malaria. Although disease accounted for more than two-thirds of all hospital admissions, the average annual disease admission rate for Vietnam (351 per 1,000 per year) was approximately one-third of that for the China-Burma-India and Southwest Pacific theaters in World War II, and more than 40 percent less than the rate for the Korean War.

Malaria was the most significant medical problem in Vietnam, but it was one which the Army Medical Department had anticipated. Studies undertaken in South America and elsewhere in Southeast Asia after World War II showed that chloroquine-resistant malaria would emerge as a problem in Vietnam. This proved to be the case in 1965, when U.S. troops began operating in the Central Highlands where there had been no real malaria eradication program because of Vietcong domination.

The precipitous rise in the incidence of *P. falciparum* malaria among combat troops in contact with the Vietcong indicated that the standard chloroquine-primaquine prophylaxis was not completely effective against this strain of plasmodium. It became apparent that another antimalarial was needed. Medical researchers concluded that DDS (4,4′-diaminodiphenylsulfone), a drug long used in the treatment of leprosy, seemed to be the most promising of many drugs under evaluation. Following intensive field tests on a priority basis in-country, it was found that the daily use of 25 milligrams of DDS, in addition to the standard chloroquine-primaquine weekly tablet, reduced the incidence of malaria by approximately one-half. This, therefore, became the operational regimen, and is now followed in tactical units operating in malaria risk areas in Vietnam.

Not only did the use of DDS, in conjunction with other antimalarials, reduce the incidence of malaria, but it also assisted greatly in lowering the incidence of relapse from a former high of almost 40 percent to a low of only 3 percent. Of equal importance, DDS aided in reducing the period of hospitalization by one-half, thus making it feasible to hold virtually all malaria patients in-country until fully recovered.

Infectious hepatitis did not pose a major problem. The incidence of this disease had been relatively low, and the disease in Vietnam was milder than in previous military experience. When the use of ISG (immune serum globulin) to provide passive immunity was instituted in mid-1964, the incidence of the disease had already begun to decline from the 1962–63 experience.

In 1964, when there were relatively few U.S. troops in Vietnam, ISG was administered to all incoming troops as a precautionary measure. For both economic and medical reasons, the dose of ISG was reduced in early 1966, and in March of that year the program was further changed to administer ISG selectively to personnel on high-risk assignments or in key positions. No major problems developed from this change in policy and procedure. The lesson here is, of course, that all decisions must be evaluated constantly and changed with boldness and courage if the situation so dictates.

The exotic tropical diseases, endemic and epidemic in Southeast Asia, did not pose a problem in U.S. troops. Plague in the Vietnamese civilian population pointed up, however, the shifting of disease patterns when the normal way of life of any peoples whose structure, economically or environmentally, is altered. Vietnam is a rice-producing and rice-exporting country. Normally, the grain flowed from the rice bowls of the interior to the few major ports of the country. The rodents which infest the areas followed the path of the rice to the ports. There they were controlled; thus, the danger of a serious outbreak of plague was averted. During the war when, for economic reasons, the South Vietnamese began to import grain, a reverse situation was created. The rice was shipped from the ports into the countryside; the rodents followed the flow of the grain inland and created havoc in the form of increased incidence of plague among the native population in areas which had heretofore been relatively free of the disease.

Contrary to experience in recent wars, neuropsychiatric illness did not constitute a significant problem. Until 1970, the rate and types of neuropsychiatric illness approximated those in the continental United States. This relatively low incidence may be attributed to the type of tactical operations being conducted; the high caliber and morale of the soldiers manning combat units; the 1-year tour; magnificent leadership; and an aggressive and effective preventive medicine program with strong command support.

However, during the wind-down in 1970, the incidence of neuropsychiatric disorders among troops increased and has remained at a disconcerting level. This increase also parallels the incidence in the United States, and has been somewhat compounded by the allegations so frequently voiced in the news media that the citizens of this country are dissatisfied with the war and the U.S. involvement therein. As the United States continues to disengage, this problem will continue, although it is known that the command, at every level, recognizes the problem and is exercising vigorous leadership to overcome it.

Combat Casualties

The wounded soldier in Vietnam received better care more quickly than in any previous conflict. This was possible because, early in the war, it was found that relatively small numbers of helicopters with an exclusive medical mission could evacuate large numbers of patients to centrally located medical facilities. As the years went by, equipment was updated, more powerful helicopters were used as air ambulances, radio communications were refined to assure more rapid response to requests for casualty evacuation, and air ambulance crews were given sufficient basic medical training to enable them to evaluate a patient's condition, to recommend the most suitable destination, and to provide resuscitative care en route. Thus, the care given to combat casualties was the finest furnished by any army to date, despite the seriousness of the wounds and the impediments to evacuation and surgical treatment.

Regardless of the criteria used—survival rates, case fatality rates, return-to-duty rates, length of hospital stay, and so forth—the Vietnam experience compares favorably with all military medical experience to date. Important factors which contributed to this record are: rapid, reliable helicopter evacuation, as noted above; well-equipped stable forward hospitals; well-trained, dedicated surgical and support teams; improved management; and continuous availability of whole blood. The availability of whole blood, which had been a problem early in each major war to date, was not a problem in Vietnam. An efficient blood distribution system kept pace with the increasing requirements for whole blood; in no instance was blood unavailable when, where, and in the types and amounts needed. The Military Blood Program Agency must be retained during peacetime and must be prepared for activation in war.

Two circumstances make this record even more remarkable. While the distribution between high velocity and fragment wounds in Vietnam approximated that of World War II and Korea, the incidence of mine and boobytrap wounds was more than triple that in the other two wars. These injuries, often multiple, always devastating, pose the most formidable threat to life and the greatest challenge to the surgeon. The helicopter contributed to survivability by delivering to hospitals greater numbers of more seriously wounded than in any war to date. These casualties included many with wounds that in past wars proved fatal before the casualty could be evacuated to a treatment facility. Despite these two factors, the survival rate remained high.

Hospitalization

Hospital support was ample for the task, both quantitatively and qualitatively. Semipermanent hospitals, located in base areas, with the most sophisticated equipment, with air-conditioned surgical and recovery suites and intensive care wards, permitted the application of the latest techniques of modern medicine in the forward battle area. Procedures that were rarely performed in the combat zone in previous wars were done on a routine daily basis in all hospitals in Vietnam.

Longer term care for patients suffering from malaria and hepatitis, or recuperating from surgery, was also provided in-country. The convalescent center at Cam Ranh Bay was used to oversee the reconditioning of the longer term patients. Availability of this convalescent center, as well as the excellent Army Medical Department facilities in Japan for those patients who could not be accommodated in Vietnam—not because facilities were not available, but rather because it was always necessary to maintain a fairly substantial number of empty beds for possible peak influx of patients—assured the command as a whole, and thus the American people, that casualties of all types who did not require onward evacuation to the continental United States, could receive all of the care necessary. Upon recovery, these men could be expeditiously returned to their units, in-country, to carry on with their assigned duties, thus conserving manpower in the theater of operations.

Environmental control within the hospital was clearly demonstrated as essential to proper military medical practice. The MUST (Medical Unit, Self-contained, Transportable) was a practical answer to control in a mobile situation. The MUST is a good concept, and Vietnam was the right war for its employment; however, there were some management deficiencies in its utilization. The MUST should have been used to establish an immediate treatment facility in new areas of operations, then replaced by less expensive semipermanent hospitals when the continuing need became apparent and construction support became available. This was not done, and the "T" (transportability) capability was not exploited.

The adequacy of hospitalization, in-country and offshore, was evidenced by the favorable survival and return-to-duty rates in both areas. The efficiency of hospitalization was greatly enhanced by effective Army and Air Force aeromedical evacuation and by a smoothly functioning medical regulating system.

Many people and many elements were responsible for the excellent record achieved in the care and treatment of the soldiers in Vietnam. The judicious and bold use of hospital facilities was certainly a major facet in this success—"bold," since hospitals in Vietnam were actually assigned missions beyond their normal TOE capabilities. Evacuation and field hospitals really functioned as 400-bed general hospitals. The 30-day evacuation policy plus the relative stability of hospitals, made possible in large measure by the outstanding in-country evacuation system, combined to permit sophisticated procedures and contributed to a high return-to-duty rate in-country.

In essence, hospitalization in Vietnam combined that normally found in the communications zone in a classic theater of operations with that found in the combat zone.

Helicopter Evacuation

Army Medical Department helicopter evacuation, in addition to moving casualties swiftly and comfortably from the battlefield to supporting hospitals, proved to be an important tool of modern military medical management. Adequate and reliable medical helicopter evacuation, with a medical radio network and an efficient medical regulating system, permitted more efficient and more economical use of medical resources.

With helicopter evacuation, hospitals can be stabilized for more efficient operation, without losing responsiveness to changing tactical situations. Hospitals need not be moved so often, with expensive "down-time" and loss of continuous support. The flexibility and versatility of helicopter evacuation under medical regulation and control permits the utilization of all the hospitals all of the time. Surgical lags are reduced. It is no longer necessary to staff every hospital with every specialty, because the casualty can be directed to that hospital best suited for the special attention he needs. At the same time, a specialty surgical capability is placed in direct support of every forward medical activity. Fewer hospitals and fewer professional personnel are required for a given operation, owing to the medical management inherent in such evacuation system as that developed in Vietnam. Despite the cost of helicopter procurement, operation, and maintenance, a *medical system* which includes helicopters is just as economical as one without helicopters, when the total costs in national resources are considered.

Tactical and strategic aeromedical evacuation support of the Army by the Air Force was magnificent and contributed in large measure to the effectiveness of the Army medical operations. The enthusiastic responsiveness of the Air Force and its ability to move large numbers of patients rapidly, on short notice, made it possible for in-country hospitals to maintain a higher bed occupancy rate in the interest of conservation of strength, without sacrificing the capacity to accommodate waves of casualties. Generally, the Air Force moved patients between larger hospitals along the coast and offshore; however, it also evacuated casualties directly from forward brigade and division bases, when requested to do so.

Similarly, there was enthusiastic cross-service support among Air Force, Navy, and Army medical facilities, in-country and offshore, as promulgated in Joint Chiefs of Staff Publication No. 3. U.S. Navy hospital ships provided invaluable augmentation to shore-based medical facilities, especially in the I Corps Tactical Zone. Interservice medical co-operation was outstanding.

Medical Supply

Medical supply support for the U.S. Army in Vietnam was superb, considering the many problems and impediments encountered. Early in the war, there was much criticism of medical supply, and a major reorganization of the existing system was required to provide adequate support. (*See Chapter V.*) It was again demonstrated, and most forcibly, that medical supply is part of the over-all medical support system, and that it must remain in that system, under professional medical control, if it is to be effective.

In addition to the existence of an unsatisfactory medical materiel management system in 1965–66, certain medical supply problems were iatrogenic ("caused by the physician").

For example, early in the buildup, it was decided to upgrade the capabilities of all hospitals in-country, because of the stability that was available and the remoteness of the objective area from the nearest offshore support. Essentially, the evacuation and field hospitals functioned as small general hospitals, and the surgical hospitals were similarly upgraded. The TOE's of these hospitals were inadequate for the expanded missions. Specialty oriented physicians immediately required different and more sophisticated types of surgical, X-ray, laboratory, and recovery and ward equipment. The impact of these requirements on medical supply and maintenance support is obvious. Also, in late 1965, medical authorities decided to add the daily DDS tablet to the weekly chloroquine-primaquine tablet in the chemoprophylaxis against *falciparum* malaria. That decision immediately created "a serious medical supply shortage" that was felt throughout the system including the manufacturer.

The wisdom of these and other operational decisions in improving the medical care in Vietnam is documented in this monograph. Medical supply was never accepted as a constraint to medical capabilities planning, and the system responded in a commendable manner.

Outpatients

All the hospitals in Vietnam were inundated with outpatients referred for specialized consultation by physicians in troop dispensaries and divisional medical activities. These hospitals were not staffed or equipped to accommodate this unprogramed workload. Adequate facilities to house and feed the referrals were usually not available; and significant discipline, control, and transportation problems arose.

The thrust of modern medical education contributed significantly to the difficulty. Many of the physicians on duty in Vietnam had come directly from civilian practice or training. Modern medical school curricula place increased emphasis on specialization and the use of specialist consultants. The sophistication of modern medicine, the desire of the physician to provide the very best care for his patient, and the increasing awareness of malpractice suits added further to the problem.

A twofold approach to resolving this problem is underway. The new modular combat support hospital, which is intended to replace the surgical and evacuation hospitals, will have a realistic outpatient capability. Of more importance, in restructuring the medical service support within the division, consideration is being given to including certain specialists in the medical battalion. Thus, outpatient consultant capability in such specialties as internal medicine, dermatology, ophthalmology, and orthopedic surgery will be available in the division base, preventing the unnecessary evacuation of many patients and keeping the troops under division control. These specialists will consult freely with other division medical officers and will also teach and visit dispensaries. In the interest of economy and mobility, division medical facilities for inpatient specialist care will not be augmented.

Battalion Surgeons

Vietnam, and other recent experience in division and brigade medical support, has shown that it is no longer necessary nor desirable to assign medical officers to combat battalions. The impact of helicopter evacuation, frequently overflying battalion aid stations and going directly to supporting medical facilities, is only one of the considerations. Equally important is the nature of modern medical education and modern medicine, and the orientation of today's young physician, who depends heavily on laboratory and X-ray facilities, and on consultations with other physicians. This is the best way to practice medicine and field medical organization is being modified to accommodate this reality.

The battalion surgeon is being removed from the combat battalion. His clinical replacement will be a well-qualified technician, probably in the grade of warrant officer, and modeled after the "physician's assistant" in civilian practice. The technician will work under the direction of physicians in the brigade base and will provide initial resuscitation to wounded and do screening at sick call. The general practice of medicine will be moved from the battalion to the brigade base.

Impact of Policies

The 1-year tour of duty, unique to the Vietnam experience, had a definite impact on the medical support system. The favorable effect of the 1-year tour on morale and the reduction of neuropsychiatric illness has been described. A more subtle effect has been on the traditional emphasis placed by the medics, and the line, on "conserving the fighting strength." Contrary to U.S. experience in conventional "open ended" or "duration plus six months" wars, this emphasis seems to have diminished in Vietnam. The political and military wisdom of certain personnel policies on evacuation and return to duty implemented in Vietnam is obvious, and the medical service must be prepared to modify its approach accordingly.

Patients medically qualified for return to duty from offshore hospitals, but with less than 60 days remaining on their Vietnam tour, were not sent back to Vietnam. Those received in offshore hospitals with less than 60 days to DEROS (date eligible for return from overseas) were further evacuated to the continental United States when the medical condition permitted. This practice lowered the return-to-duty rates and the workloads of the various hospitals in the chain of evacuation. Approximately one-sixth of the patients evacuated offshore were administratively ineligible to return to duty in Vietnam, regardless of the medical condition or the degree of recovery. This reason, among others, contributed to the decision to have a 60-day offshore evacuation policy, rather than the traditional 120-day holding policy.

This "60 days remaining on DEROS" policy was also one of the factors responsible for the increase of the in-country holding policy from 15 to 30 days. (There are other more cogent ones.) The increased capability and holding capacity of in-country hospitals led to more selective evacuation of complicated cases, largely surgical, to the offshore hospitals in Japan and elsewhere. Patients with simple surgical, medical, and neuropsychiatric ailments were treated in-country and returned to duty there. The imbalance between the types of patients received offshore, and the balanced staff prepared to receive them, created a management problem. Repeatedly, the Army was challenged on "under utilization" of offshore capability by "managers" who could not understand why a 1,000-bed general hospital was "full" with only 650 patients. In fact, a 1,000-bed general hospital, staffed for a 40–40–20 percent mix of medical, surgical, and neuropsychiatric patients, was inundated with 650 patients, most of whom required complicated surgery, often orthopedic.

A more insidious policy, which troubled me as a physician and staff officer, was the provision that patients evacuated to the continental United States, or home of record, would be given tour-completion credit and would not be required to return to Vietnam. Originally the policy applied to battle wounded only, but later it also included disease and nonbattle injury cases. This expansion of the policy gave me the most concern, because it damaged the safety and preventive medicine programs by giving a bonus to the careless or disaffected manipulator. There was a time, in the fall of 1965, when the best way for a soldier to insure being home with his family on Christmas was to contract malaria in the Highlands, or to be seriously injured in a Honda accident in Saigon, or to receive a bad "accidental" burn in Nha Trang. At the subconscious level, where a soldier is really motivated, such a bonus in illness or injury can have a most negative effect.

In late 1968, USARV made extraordinary efforts to meet in-country strength ceilings imposed by higher authority. Although the so-called "patient account" portion of the USARV troop strength was established at 3,500, the surgeon was directed to reduce the number of patients occupying beds to no more than 3,000, to provide spaces to cover accesses in in-country temporary duty personnel. Also, some 5,000 hospital beds were available during that period. There seemed to be little command concern about the overevacuation offshore to accomplish the reduction. In fact, when informed that certain patients who would be fit for return to duty within, say, 5 days, were being evacuated to Japan one senior commander said that he sent troops to Japan for only 5 days on a recurrent basis—the R&R (rest and recuperation) Program. In short, there seemed to be less command concern in retaining experienced combat troops in-country, because of the ready availability of replacements.

These observations are not intended to be critical, but they should be considered when developing future policy related to eligibility to return to combat zones after illness or injury. Modifications of Medical Department policy and procedure, and the allocation of resources among successive medical treatment echelons, must also be done in light of these realities.

Lack of Responsiveness of The Army Authorization Document System

A major problem encountered in the buildup phase was the lack of responsiveness to TAADS (The Army Authorization Document System) in the combat situation. When the decision was made in 1965 to upgrade the capabilities of in-country hospitals, their TOE's were grossly inadequate for the expanded missions. Authorizations for the additional personnel and equipment required were hopelessly delayed, first by the moratorium in effect on TAADS, then by the inertia of the system. The most frustrating part of the problem was securing authorizations against which to requisition nonmedical equipment and enlisted personnel (including medical).

Through the use of effective technical channels, The Surgeon General most expeditiously provided the Medical Department officers and the medical equipment needed for the expanded hospital missions. Enlisted personnel and the nonmedical equipment, however, had to be processed through nonmedical channels, involving months of delay.

While TAADS may be an effective way to manage force structure in peacetime, it should be waived in the combat situation to permit timely implementation of decisions necessary to support operations.

Research

Clinical research, surgical and medical, in forward combat hospitals, essential to the finest practice of medicine and to the improvement of technique and materiel procedures, was done most effectively in Vietnam. Adequate photographic as well as written documentation of combat medical experience was also furnished for review and evaluation in the refinement of procedures.

Vietnamese Civilian Care

While providing the best in medical care for U.S. forces, the Medical Department made significant contributions to the care of sick and injured Vietnamese civilians from the earliest days of U.S. involvement. These efforts, of considerable magnitude and scope, were well integrated with other United States and Vietnamese efforts and contributed to the improvement of Vietnamese medical practices.

Despite frequent and continuing political allegations to the contrary, U.S. troops were compassionate and did provide full assistance to the disrupted Vietnamese nation. Apart from the humanitarian aspects of the various civilian medical assistance programs, this involvement provided U.S. medical personnel gainful and rewarding activity during lulls between peak military medical support requirements. This, in turn, contributed to the high morale of committed U.S. "medics."

Civilian Implications

In every major war, medical advances are made which have a strong positive influence on the over-all practice of medicine in civilian society. Vietnam was no exception. Skilled surgical and research teams developed improved techniques for managing trauma in individuals and in groups. Examples of specific advances are contained in the body of this monograph. Less obvious is the tremendous contribution that physicians and surgeons are making to American medicine as a result of their in-depth experience in Vietnam. Throughout the Nation, there are young surgeons completely competent to handle the most complicated and serious of injuries, whether due to accident, natural disaster, or war. Similarly, physicians returning to their civilian practices bring with them diagnostic and therapeutic capability to manage the most baffling and complicated medical conditions. No other country in the world is so blessed.

Improved medical management, developed on the field of battle, has direct application in civilian practice. Regionalization of medical care delivery and increased utilization of ancillary health care personnel under the team concept, now receiving so much attention at national and local levels, are patterned on the military model that has been used for many years. The medical control concept, medical radio network and helicopter evacuation—the systems approach which proved so successful in Vietnam—is now being used for efficient, effective regionalized health care delivery in the United States.

The highly successful MAST (Military Assistance to Safety in Traffic) Program is but one prime example of the adaptation of the military model to the civilian requirement. This demonstration project cannot help but expand, and the hope is that before too long the civilian community, rural and metropolitan, may achieve a real emergency medical care system approaching the effectiveness of that provided in Vietnam. The Vietnam veteran, having seen what can be done half way around the world, is now demanding that the same capability be provided here at home.

As in previous wars, the medical experience gained in Vietnam is likely to contribute to the saving of more lives in the future than were lost during the conflict.

This, then, is the story of the medical support of the U.S. Army in Vietnam. The challenge was met with vigor and enthusiasm, and the mission was accomplished in the highest tradition of the U.S. Army and its Medical Department.

Glossary

ACofS	Assistant Chief of Staff
Adj	Adjutant
Admin	Administration, administrative, administrator
Adv	Adviser
AID	United States Agency for International Development
Amb	Ambulance
AMSC	Army Medical Specialist Corps
ANC	Army Nurse Corps
AR	Army regulation
ARVN	Army Republic of Vietnam
ASWBPL	Armed Services Whole Blood Processing Laboratory
ATTLEBORO	Operation resulting in a battle that took place in September–November 1966 northwest of Saigon. Over 22,000 American and South Vietnamese troops defeated the Viet Cong 9th Division, reinforced by a North Vietnamese regiment, and drove them back to the Cambodian border.
Average strength	Arithmetic mean (average) of daily morning report strengths, used in medical statistical reports for computing admission rates, mortality rates, and noneffective rates
CBI	China-Burma-India theater (World War II)
CG	Commanding general
CINCPAC	Commander in Chief, Pacific
CINCUSARPAC	Commander in Chief, U.S. Army, Pacific
Civ	Civilian
Comdr	Commander
Comm	Communications
COMUSMACV	Commander, United States Military Assistance Command, Vietnam
Con	Consul, consulate
CONEX	Container express
CONUS	Continental United States
COSTAR	Combat service to the Army study

CRO	Carded for record only. Pertaining to medical cases not treated on an "excused from duty" status, but of sufficient seriousness or of sufficient potential medical or administrative interest that individual medical records are required to be prepared in the same manner as for "excused from duty" cases
CTZ	Corps tactical zone
CWCP	Civilian War Casualty Program
DBC	Deputy brigade commander
DC	Dental Corps
DCG	Deputy commanding general
DCS	Deputy Chief of Staff
DDS	Diaminodiphenylsulfone
Den	Dental
DENTCAP	Dental Civic Action Program (dental counterpart to MEDCAP)
DEROS	Date eligible for return from overseas
DSA	Defense Supply Agency
Dust-off	Army medical evacuation helicopter units not organic to divisions
ExecO	Executive officer
FASCOM	A field army support command
FEJMRO	Far East Medical Regulating Office
FEST	Field Epidemiologic Survey Team
FUO	Fever of undetermined origin
FWMAF	Free World Military Assistance Forces
G–1	Assistant Chief of Staff for Personnel
G–4	Assistant Chief of Staff for Logistics
IBM	International Business Machines
IHS	Idiopathic Hemorrhagic Syndrome
Intel	Intelligence
ISG	Immune serum globulin
KIA	Killed in action
LST	Landing ship, tank
MAAGV	United States Military Assistance Advisory Group, Vietnam
MAST	Military Assistance to Safety in Traffic
MBPA	Military Blood Program Agency
MC	Medical Corps
MEDCAP	Medical Civic Action Program
Med Mat	Medical materiel
Mgt	Management

Mil Med	Military medicine
MILPHAP	Military Provincial Health Assistance Program
Mob	Mobile
MOS	Military occupational specialty
MPR	Military pay record
Mpr Con	Manpower control
MRO	Medical regulating office(r)
MSC	Medical Service Corps
MUST	Medical unit, self-contained, transportable
NAMRU	Naval Medical Research Unit
NCR	National Cash Register
Opns	Operations
P&A	Personnel and administration
PACOM	Pacific Command
Pers	Personnel
PF	Popular Forces
PHAP	Provincial Health Assistance Program
PIO	Public information office(r)
Pol	Policies
POW	Prisoner of war
Prev Med	Preventive medicine
Prof Svc	Professional service
PSC	Personnel service company
Reg	Regulating, regulator
RF	Regional Forces
ROAD	Reorganization Objective Army Divisions
R&R	Rest and recuperation
RVN	The Republic of Vietnam
RVNAF	Republic of Vietnam Armed Forces
S-1	Adjutant (U.S. Army)
S-3	Operations and training officer (U.S. Army)
S-4	Supply officer (U.S. Army)
Sch	School
Sci	Science
Scty	Security
SEATO	Southeast Asia Treaty Organization
Sec	Section
Stat	Statistics
SWPA	Southwest Pacific theater (World War II)
TAADS	The Army Authorization Document System
TASTA	The administrative support theater Army
TCP	Tropical Canine Pancytopenia
Tng	Training

TOE	Table of organization and equipment
USAMEDCOMV	United States Army Medical Command, Vietnam (Provisional)
USAMMA	United States Army Medical Materiel Agency
USAMRDC	United States Army Medical Research and Development Command
USARPAC	United States Army, Pacific
USARV	United States Army, Vietnam
USARYIS	United States Army, Ryukyu Islands
USASCV	United States Army Support Command, Vietnam
USASGV	United States Army Support Group, Vietnam
USDA	United States Department of Agriculture
USMACV	United States Military Assistance Command, Vietnam
USOM	United States Operations Mission
USPHS	United States Public Health Service
Vet	Veterinary, veterinarian
VETCAP	Veterinary Civic Action Program (veterinary part of MEDCAP)
WIA	Wounded in action
WRAIR	Walter Reed Army Institute of Research

Index

Made in United States
Cleveland, OH
06 November 2026

47678359R10114